Student Workbook for

THE ADMINISTRATIVE DENTAL ASSISTANT

Fourth Edition

Linda J. Gaylor, RDA, BPA, MEd
Coordinator, Curriculum and Instruction
San Bernardino County Superintendent of Schools
Regional Occupational Program, Career Training, and Support Services
San Bernardino, California

ELSEVIER

ELSEVIER

3251 Riverport Lane
St. Louis, Missouri 63043

ISBN: 978-0-3232-9451-5

STUDENT WORKBOOK FOR THE ADMINISTRATIVE DENTAL ASSISTANT, FOURTH EDITION

Notices

Knowledge and best practice in this field are constantly changing. As new research and experience broaden our understanding, changes in research methods, professional practices, or medical treatment may become necessary.

Practitioners and researchers must always rely on their own experience and knowledge in evaluating and using any information, methods, compounds, or experiments described herein. In using such information or methods they should be mindful of their own safety and the safety of others, including parties for whom they have a professional responsibility.

With respect to any drug or pharmaceutical products identified, readers are advised to check the most current information provided (i) on procedures featured or (ii) by the manufacturer of each product to be administered, to verify the recommended dose or formula, the method and duration of administration, and contraindications. It is the responsibility of practitioners, relying on their own experience and knowledge of their patients, to make diagnoses, to determine dosages and the best treatment for each individual patient, and to take all appropriate safety precautions.

To the fullest extent of the law, neither the Publisher nor the authors, contributors, or editors assume any liability for any injury and/or damage to persons or property as a matter of products liability, negligence or otherwise, or from any use or operation of any methods, products, instructions, or ideas contained in the material herein.

Content Strategist: Kristin Wilhelm
Content Development Manager: Ellen Wurm-Cutter
Associate Content Development Specialist: Katie Gutierrez
Publishing Services Manager: Hemamalini Rajendrababu
Project Manager: Manchu Mohan
Cover Designer: Muthukumaran Thangaraj

Printed in the United States of America

Last digit is the print number: 9 8 7 6 5 4 3 2 1

Working together
to grow libraries in
developing countries

www.elsevier.com • www.bookaid.org

Introduction

The Student Workbook, DVD-ROM, and Evolve companion website have been designed to help you perfect the skills and objectives presented in *The Administrative Dental Assistant*, fourth edition. To help you achieve these objectives, this workbook includes the following features:

- An **Introduction** briefly states the key concept and goals of each chapter.
- **Learning Objectives** identify the concepts and skills that are necessary to master the goal of each chapter.
- **Exercises** ask questions that require you to list information, identify key concepts, and match terms with their definitions. Short-answer questions direct you to solve problems and sequence activities. These exercises are intended to help you achieve the objectives in the textbook by providing a means by which you can study, work with others, and develop necessary skills.
- **Activity Exercises** help you apply information learned to complete tasks that are similar to tasks you will encounter as an administrative dental assistant. The activities require you to use information assembled in one activity to complete the next task. It is very important that you complete the tasks in the order in which they are presented. Before moving on to the next task, you should verify the correctness of the completed task. Referring to information identified in the "Anatomy of..." figures and procedures outlined in the textbook may prove helpful. *Remember:* The tasks are sequenced and must be completed in the order presented.
- **Dentrix Exercises** introduce you to a *real-world* dental practice management software and are designed to help develop basic skills. Dentrix is a leader in dental practice management software and dental office technology integration. The DVD provided in this workbook is the Dentrix Learning Edition, a special version of Dentrix G4 designed specifically for educational purposes. It includes a preloaded database of patients and is interactive, allowing you to perform various tasks the way they are done in a dental office. The accompanying *User's Guide* walks you through all the tasks and functions of the program and provides an opportunity for you to explore more advanced functions of the dental practice management software.
- **Dental Practice Procedural Manual Project** is an optional project that provides a way for you to *practice* various Career Ready Practices, such as collaboration, teamwork, critical thinking, communications, and application of technical skills. By working on this project, which spans the full textbook, your team will do research, have discussions, and come to consensus about the information you will include in your procedural manual. The majority of the information your team will need will be in the textbook and created during the Career Ready Practices exercises at the end of each chapter.
- The companion Evolve website for *The Administrative Dental Assistant* was created specifically to help enhance the experiences of both students and instructors using the textbook and workbook. Accessible via http://evolve.elsevier.com/Gaylor/ada, the following resources are provided:
- Practice Quizzes
- Image Collection
- Career Ready Practice Grading Rubrics

Plus...
"Day in the Life" Simulation Tool
The features of this interactive software are designed to guide you through simulated tasks typical to a dental business office. For each day of the week in the program, the level of difficulty is increased and new concepts are introduced. Concepts are directly related to material in the textbook. On later days of the week you will be required to independently apply information and concepts that you have learned in the textbook. You may find the exercises to have more significance after completing Chapters 3 through 17.

The interactive program simulates a "Day in the Life of an Administrative Dental Assistant" and challenges you to complete tasks as they would occur in the workplace, such as organizing functions, prioritizing tasks, solving problems, and completing daily tasks typical of an administrative dental assistant. Exam and study modes incorporated into the program provide flexibility in teaching and learning. Whereas the exam mode requires you to log in and complete the tasks in order from Monday through Friday, tracking your progress and outputting a results sheet, the study mode allows you to enter any day and time throughout the weeklong exercise to practice or review specific procedures.

- A variety of tasks typical in practice management software are included: entering and updating patient data, posting payment and treatment procedures, submitting insurance e-claims for payment, evaluating reports, and scheduling appointments.
- Patients arrive for appointments, and you must complete related tasks such as updating patient information and completing the checkout process. The mail arrives on a daily basis and must be processed. The telephone rings, and you must take care of the caller.
- Pop-ups ask you questions about a particular subject relevant to the task at hand. Prompts indicate whether you have answered each question correctly or incorrectly and provide a rationale. (You can go back and view the correct response if you have answered incorrectly.)

I hope that you will find the textbook and the accompanying material useful in pursuing an exciting career as a member of a dental healthcare team.

Linda J. Gaylor

Reviewers

Jamie Collins RDH, CDA
Dental Assisting Educator
Business Partnership/Workforce Development—Dental Assisting
College of Western Idaho
Nampa, Idaho

Joseph W. Robertson, DDS, BS
Faculty
Department of Nursing and Health Professions
Oakland Community College
Bloomfield Hills, Michigan

Contents

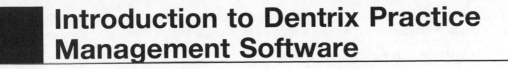

Introduction to Dentrix Practice Management Software

These steps have been prepared to help minimize or eliminate any issues when installing the Dentrix Learning Edition. For a successful installation, follow the steps below exactly. Please read through all the steps before attempting to install the Learning Edition.

1. Ensure System Meets the System Requirements

For optimal performance with the Learning Edition, it is important to review the system requirements and make sure your system can accommodate them before you install the Learning Edition. The Dentrix Learning Edition system requirements are available at www.dentrix.com/training/dentrix-learning-edition.aspx. Please be aware of the following:

■ The Dentrix Learning Edition runs on a Windows platform and can run on only Microsoft Windows XP or higher.

■ The computer's graphics card may need to be upgraded to take advantage of the 3-D modeling features in the Learning Edition.

■ Adequate processor speed is important to help reduce or eliminate any latency/performance issues as they relate to the Learning Edition. The amount of free memory on the computer can greatly impact the performance of the computer and also the performance of the overall Dentrix system. Reducing or eliminating the number of unnecessary processes on a computer can significantly improve a computer's performance.

When the system requirements are closely scrutinized and adhered to, the potential for a successful installation experience increases dramatically.

2. Check Available Disk Space

From the Start menu, select My Computer and highlight the C: drive icon. Select View > Details from the menu bar, or right-click on the C: drive icon and select Properties. The Local Disk Properties dialog box appears. The General tab will display the Used and Free Disk Space.

Consult the Dentrix Learning Edition System Requirements to view the required free hard disk space for workstations. The current Dentrix system requirements are available online at www.dentrix.com/training/dentrix-learning-edition.aspx. You may experience slowness if your system does not meet the requirements for available memory or hard drive space. If your system is very deficient in memory, the Learning Edition might not be able to install on your system until you upgrade your system and get more memory.

3. Important! Close All Other Applications

Look at the Windows Notification Area (normally in the bottom right corner of the screen, near the system time) and close any programs that appear there. As with most programs, you must disable any antivirus software on the computer and the Windows screensaver for the duration of the installation. When the install is complete, enable the antivirus software and the Windows screensaver.

4. Follow the Installation Instructions

Follow the step-by-step instructions in this guide to install the Dentrix Learning Edition.

5. Finish the Installation Completely

Do not interrupt the installation process, even if it looks as though nothing is happening. You will be prompted when the installation is ready to continue. Terminating an installation prior to completion could affect the integrity of the database.

NOTE: If you are using Windows Vista, you may see messages during the installation process that are not shown in these steps. Follow the on-screen prompts for those messages as they appear and continue with the installation as directed in the steps below.

1. Insert the Dentrix Learning Edition DVD into the DVD drive. If the DVD drive is equipped with AutoStart technology, the **Dentrix G4 Install Welcome** screen appears within a few seconds (see below).

   - If you see the Welcome screen, proceed to step 2.

   - If the Welcome screen does not appear:

   a. Click the Windows **Start** button and select **Run**. The **Run** dialog box appears.

   b. Type **D:\Disk1\Setup** in the command line (where D: is the drive letter for the DVD drive). Click the **OK** button to begin the installation.

   c. Click **Install Software**. The screen that appears lists the products you can install. From this screen, you can install the Dentrix Learning Edition and the Required Components.

INSTALL SOFTWARE	IMPORTANT INSTALLATION TIPS	ADD-ON PRODUCTS	CONTACT US	CUSTOMER SERVICE	EXPLORE THIS CD

DENTRIX®

G4

INSPIRED

WELCOME TO G4

DENTRIX G4 is the next generation of premiere practice management software from Henry Schein Practice Solutions that will empower you to go farther and do more! Please read "Important Installation Tips," available from the options menu, before installing your DENTRIX G4 software.

▶ INSTALL DENTRIX G4

▶ INSTALL DXMOBILE

▶ INSTALL REQUIRED COMPONENTS

EXIT

2. Click the **Install Required Components** install option to display the Required Components information (see below). Follow the instructions below to install the required components.

INSTALL
SOFTWARE
IMPORTANT
INSTALLATION TIPS
ADD-ON
PRODUCTS
CONTACT
US
CUSTOMER
SERVICE
EXPLORE
THIS CD

DENTRIX®

G4

INSPIRED

REQUIRED COMPONENTS

These components—.NET Framework, DirectX 9.0, Windows Journal Viewer, and Crystal Reports .NET Components are required for many of the new and exciting features of DENTRIX G4 to function properly. These components will be automatically installed when you install DENTRIX G4. Select "INSTALL NOW" to launch a customized install of these components.

INSTALL NOW

▶ INSTALL DENTRIX G4

▶ INSTALL DXMOBILE

▶ INSTALL REQUIRED COMPONENTS

EXIT

a. Click **Install Now** to install the required components. The InstallShield Wizard will perform a check of your system to verify that all the required components are installed. After the InstallShield Wizard has performed the check, a screen appears with a list of the required components and whether or not they are installed on your system (see following page).

NOTE: If you already have all the required components installed, click Finish to close the Required Components install dialog box and return to the main installation screen.

Introduction to Dentrix Practice Management Software

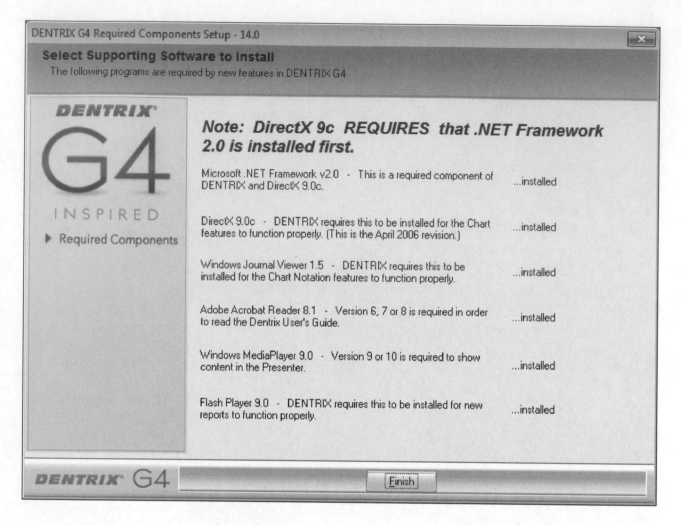

b. Click **Install All** to install all the required components. If desired, you can install each component one at a time by clicking Install next to the component, waiting for the install to finish, and clicking Install on the next component.

As components are installed, you might receive several on-screen messages or prompts. Follow the on-screen prompts to install the required components.

NOTE: If you are installing Adobe Flash Player 9, you may see an error message during the install. Click OK to the error message. If other components need to be installed, the installation continues.

c. Once all the required components have been installed, click the **Close** button (the red "X" button in the top right corner). An **Exit Setup** message appears (see below).

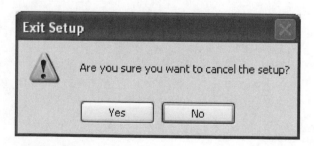

d. Click **Yes** on the Exit Setup message to indicate that you want to cancel the setup and return to the Required Components information on the main install screen.

3. Click **Install Dentrix G4**. The **Dentrix Learning Edition installation information** appears (see below).

INSTALL
SOFTWARE
IMPORTANT
INSTALLATION TIPS
ADD-ON
PRODUCTS
CONTACT
US
CUSTOMER
SERVICE
EXPLORE
THIS CD

DENTRIX ®

G4

INSPIRED

DENTRIX G4

To begin the installation of DENTRIX G4, click "INSTALL NOW" then sit back and watch as we add new features, tools, and functionality that transforms your DENTRIX system into a richer, more robust system. **Please refer to "Important Installation Tips" before** installing DENTRIX G4.

INSTALL NOW

▶ INSTALL DENTRIX G4

▶ INSTALL DXMOBILE

▶ INSTALL REQUIRED COMPONENTS

EXIT

Introduction to Dentrix Practice Management Software

4. Click the **Install Now** link at the bottom of the Dentrix Learning Edition installation information. The InstallShield Wizard loads and the **Welcome** screen appears (see below).

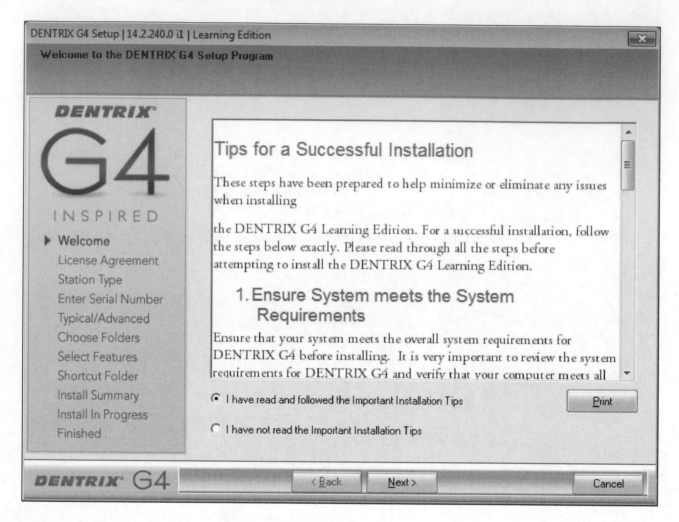

5. Read the Tips for a Successful Installation on this screen. When you have read the tips, mark **I have read and followed the tips for a successful installation** and click **Next** to continue. The **License Agreement** screen appears (see below).

   NOTE: If you want to print the Tips for a Successful Installation, click the Print button.

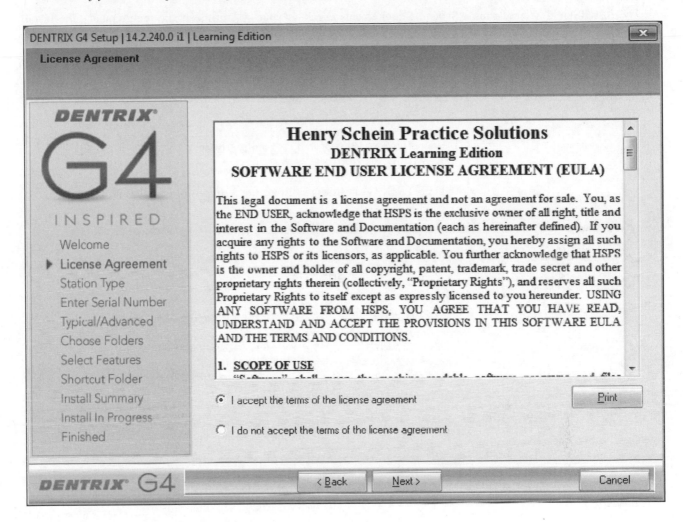

6. Read the Dentrix Learning Edition Software End User License Agreement. When you have read the document, mark **I accept the terms of the license agreement** and click **Next** to continue.

NOTE: You can print a copy of the Dentrix Learning Edition Software End User License Agreement by clicking the Print button.

The InstallShield Wizard runs a System Requirements check. If your system meets the requirements, the Install continues to step 8. If your system does not meet the requirements, the **System Requirements Notice** dialog box appears and lists the deficiencies in your system (see below).

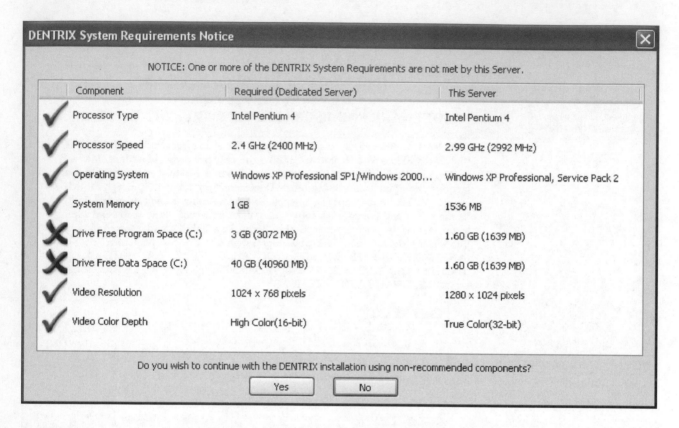

NOTE: The Learning Edition system requirements are available at www.dentrix.com/training/dentrix-learning-edition.aspx.

7. If the **System Requirements Notice** appears, verify the system requirements. A green check mark indicates that a component meets the requirements. A red "X" indicates that a component does not meet the requirements. Click **Yes** to continue the installation without meeting the recommended system requirements. The **Choose Folders** screen appears (see below).

If desired, you can click **No** to stop the installation and upgrade your system. However, that is not required for the Dentrix Learning Edition.

NOTE: The Dentrix Learning Edition may still function if your system does not meet the requirements. However, you may experience slowness if your system does not meet the requirements for available memory or hard drive space. If your system is very deficient in memory, the Learning Edition might not be able to install on your system until you upgrade your system and get more memory.

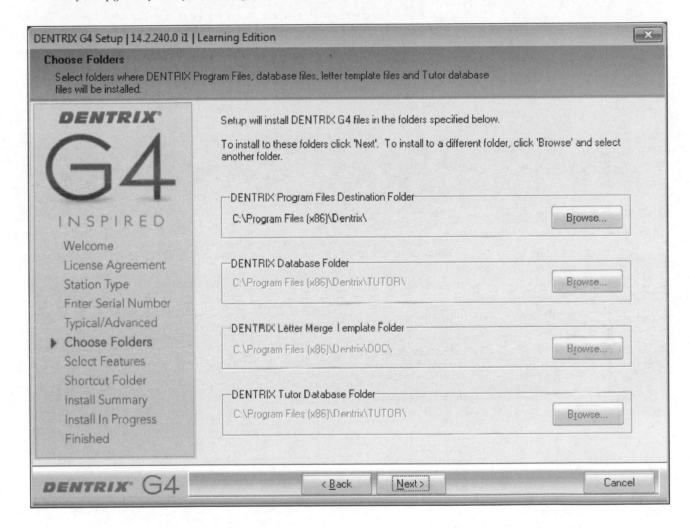

Introduction to Dentrix Practice Management Software

8. Select the folder where you want to store the Dentrix Learning Edition program files. If you do not want to store the program files in the folder that is recommended on the screen, you can select a new folder. Otherwise, leave the folder location as it is.

NOTE: The following folder locations are listed on the screen with the program files. With the Learning Edition, you can change only the location of the program files. The explanations below are for your reference only.

- *Program Files: The executable files that are required to make the program run. Your program files should be stored in the place where you want the Dentrix Learning Edition files to be stored.*

- *Database Files: The files that include your patient information files and the program settings that are specific to your office. The Tutor database is automatically set as your database.*

- *Letter Merge Templates: The Microsoft Word default letter templates that are used during the letter merge. These templates are automatically saved to the DOC folder.*

- *Tutor Database: A practice database that is used for training. These files are automatically installed.*

If you want to use the default folder location for the program files, click **Next**. If you want to change the program file folder location, click **Browse** and navigate to the desired location. The **Install Summary** screen appears (see below).

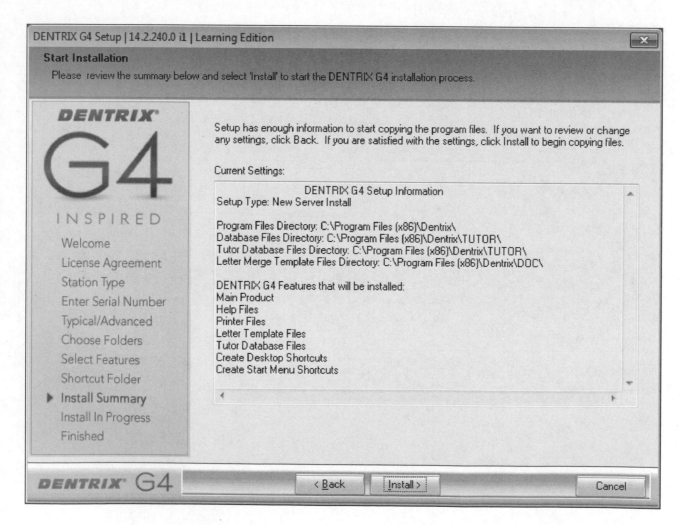

9. Click **Install** to begin installing the Dentrix Learning Edition. After a few minutes, the **Guru Limited Edition Server Installation Wizard** appears (see below).

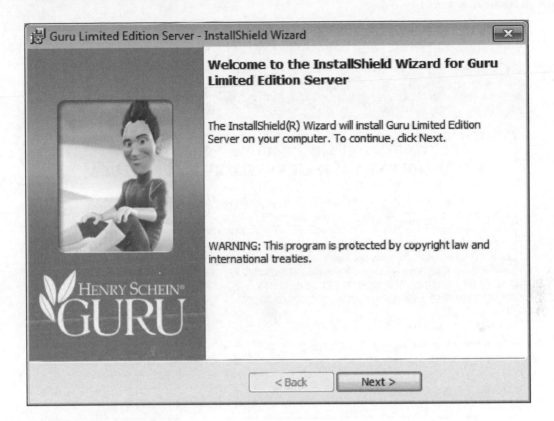

Introduction to Dentrix Practice Management Software

10. Guru Limited Edition is a patient education tool that can be accessed from the Dentrix Chart. Click **Next** on the **Guru Limited Edition Server Welcome** screen to continue with the installation. The **Guru Limited Edition license agreement** appears (see below).

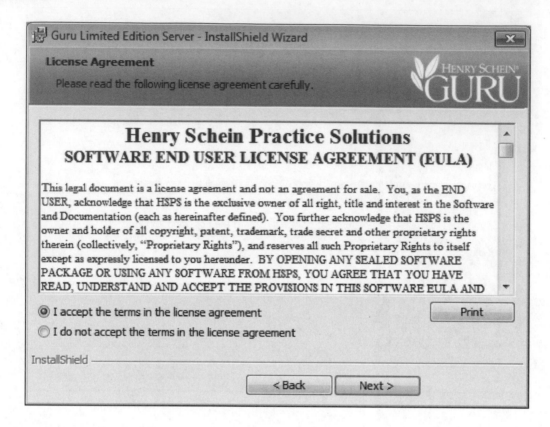

Introduction to Dentrix Practice Management Software

11. Read the Guru Limited Edition Software End User License Agreement. When you have read the document, mark **I accept the terms of the license agreement** and click **Next** to continue. The **Firewall Configuration** screen appears (see below.)

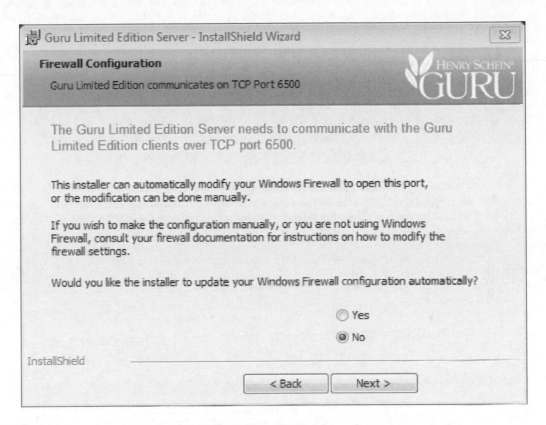

NOTE: *You can print a copy of the Guru Learning Edition Software End User License Agreement by clicking the Print button.*

12. With the commercial edition of Dentrix, the Guru Limited Edition Server needs access to a specific port in the system to function properly. Typically, this port is blocked by firewall protection.

With the Learning Edition, the Guru Limited Edition Server does not need to access this port, so you do not need to allow Guru to change your firewall configuration. Make sure **No** is selected on the **Firewall Configuration** screen. Click **Next** to continue with the installation. The **Ready to Install** screen appears (see below).

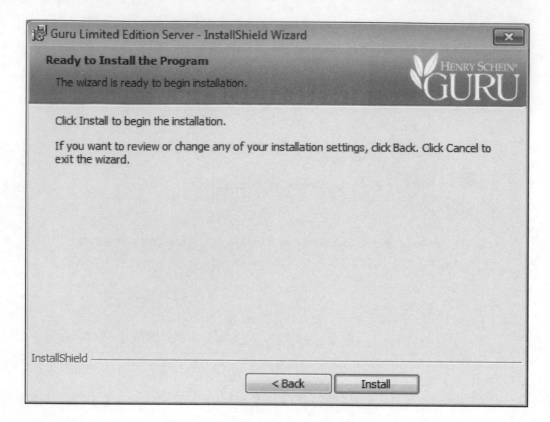

13. Click **Install** to begin the Guru Limited Edition Server installation. The **InstallShield Wizard Complete** screen appears when the install is finished (see below).

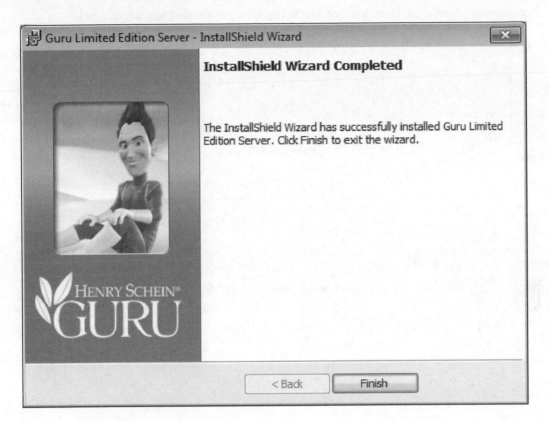

Introduction to Dentrix Practice Management Software

14. Click **Finish** to complete the Guru Limited Edition Server installation. The install continues with the rest of the Dentrix Learning Edition installation.

    After the Dentrix software has been installed, the **Setup Complete** screen appears (see below).

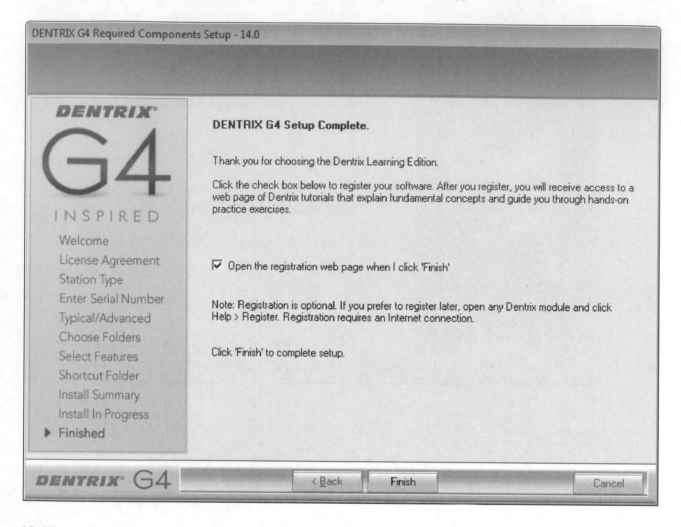

15. Un-check **Open the registration web page when I click 'Finish.'** You are not required to register your Dentrix Learning Edition software.

16. Click **Finish** to finish the Dentrix Learning Edition installation. The InstallShield Wizard will close and you will return to the **Dentrix Learning Edition installation** screen.

17. Click **Exit** to close the **Dentrix Learning Edition installation** screen. The InstallShield Wizard places six shortcuts on your Windows Desktop. These shortcuts open Dentrix modules and give you access to the Dentrix G4 User's Guide (see below).

    ■ **Appointments:** Opens the Dentrix Appointment Book, the module you use to schedule patient appointments and manage your schedule.

    ■ **Family File:** Opens the Dentrix Family File, the module you use to enter patient records and manage patient information.

    ■ **Ledger:** Opens the Dentrix Ledger, the module you use to enter payments and manage accounts.

    ■ **Office Manager:** Opens the Dentrix Office Manager, the module you use to run reports and set up practice defaults.

- **Patient Chart:** Opens the Dentrix Patient Chart, the module you use to chart treatment and enter clinical notes.

- **Dentrix Launcher:** Opens the Dentrix Launcher tool, which shows the Dentrix modules in the context of an office and helps you open the correct module for the task you want to perform.

- **Dentrix G4 User's Guide:** Opens a PDF of the Dentrix G4 User's Guide.

- **Productivity Pack 7 Update Guide:** Opens a PDF of the guide that describes the new features that were added to Dentrix G4 in Productivity Pack 7.

- **Productivity Pack 8 Update Guide:** Opens a PDF of the guide that describes the new features that were added to Dentrix G4 in Productivity Pack 8.

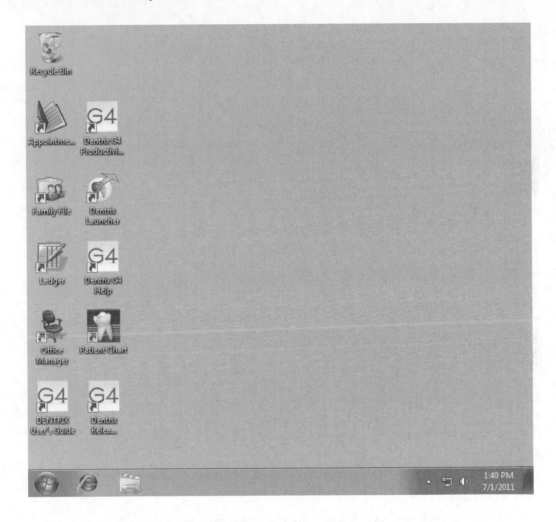

DISABLING THE ESYNC, WEBSYNC, AND PRACTICE ASSISTANT TASK MANAGER

The eSync, WebSync, and Practice Assistant Task Manager are processes that run automatically with the commercial edition of Dentrix G4. You do not need to use these processes with the Dentrix Learning Edition. It is recommended that you disable these processes to prevent them from running automatically.

If you don't disable these processes, you will receive notifications when the eSync and WebSync run automatically. If you don't disable the Practice Assistant Manager, you will receive error messages when you try to shut down your computer. Follow the instructions below to disable the eSync, WebSync, and Practice Assistant Task Manager.

Disabling the eSync

eSync is the process by which information is passed between the commercial edition of Dentrix and some of the Dentrix add-on features that are not available with the Learning Edition. It is important to disable this process and prevent it from running automatically with the Learning Edition.

NOTE: If you do not disable eSync, it will run automatically and you will receive eSync notifications daily. It is important to disable eSync to prevent it from running automatically.

The eSync setup is located in your computer's Notification Area. The eSync icon looks like a white "e" in a red circle (see below).

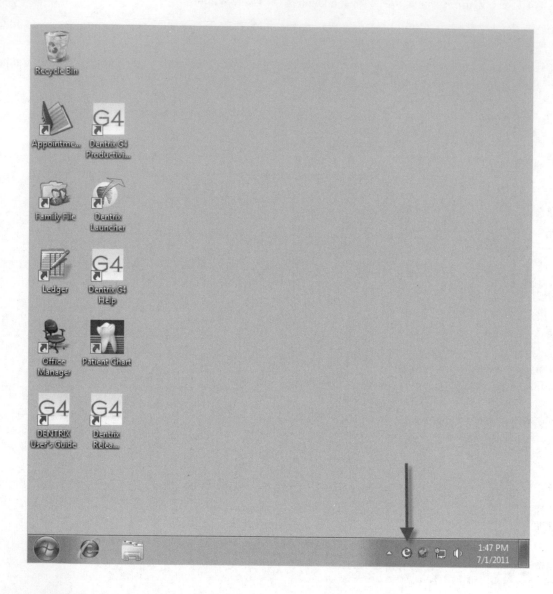

Follow the steps below to prevent the eSync from running automatically:

1. Locate the eSync icon in the Windows Notification Area. If the icon appears in the Notification Area, skip to step 2. If the icon does not appear in the Notification Area, follow steps a and b.

   a. Click the Windows **Start** button, select **All Programs**, and select **Startup** from the menu.

   b. Select **eSync Reminder** from the **Startup** menu. The **eSync** icon appears in the Notification Area.

2. Right-click the eSync icon and select **Open eSync Setup**. The **eSync Setup** dialog box appears (see below).

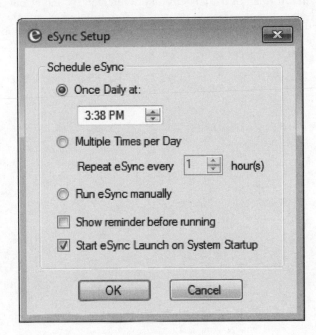

3. To prevent eSync from running automatically every day, mark **Run eSync Manually**. Do not change the other settings in the dialog box.

4. Click **OK** to the confirmation message that appears.

5. Click **OK** to close the **eSync Setup** dialog box. The eSync process is now disabled.

NOTE: eSync is set to start up each time you restart your computer and to run in the background while you work. This is beneficial for offices because they need to use the eSync functionality throughout the day. Since you do not need to use eSync, you can remove it from your Windows Startup folder and prevent it from starting up and running.

To remove eSync from your Startup folder, click the Windows **Start** button and click **All Programs**. Right-click the folder called **Startup** and click **Open All Users**. In the folder that opens, right-click the **eSync** icon, and click **Delete**. Click **Yes** to the message that appears. eSync will be deleted from the Windows Startup tasks and will not open on your computer again.

Disabling the WebSync

WebSync is the process by which information is transferred between Dentrix and eCentral with the commercial edition of Dentrix. It is important to disable this process and prevent it from running automatically with the Learning Edition.

NOTE: If you do not disable the WebSync, it will run automatically and you will receive WebSync notifications daily. It is important to disable the WebSync to prevent it from running automatically.

The WebSync Reminder icon is located in your Notification Area. The icon looks like a world with red and blue arrows around it (see below).

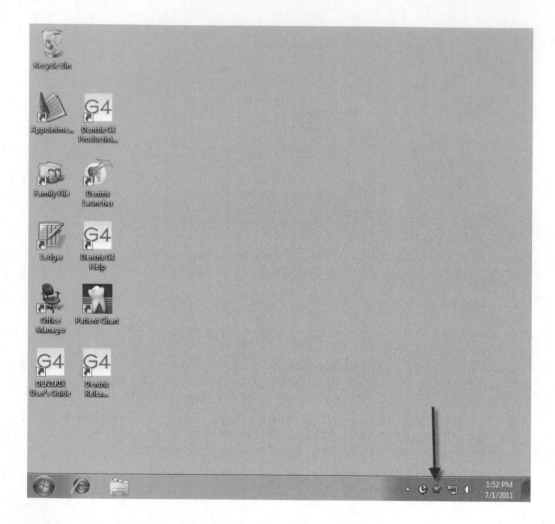

Follow the steps below to prevent WebSync from running automatically:

1. Locate the WebSync Reminder icon in the Notification Area. If the icon appears in the Notification Area, skip to step 2. If the icon does not appear in the Notification Area, follow steps a and b.

   a. Click the Windows **Start** button, select **All Programs**, and select **Startup** from the menu.

   b. Select **WebSync Reminder** from the **Startup** menu. The **WebSync Reminder** icon appears in the Notification Area.

2. Right-click the **WebSync Reminder** icon and select **Open the DXWeb Toolbar**. The **DXWeb Toolbar** appears (see below).

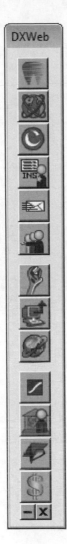

3. Click the **Settings** button (see below) and select **WebSync Wizard** from the menu.

4. Click **Next** on the **WebSync Wizard Welcome** screen (see below).

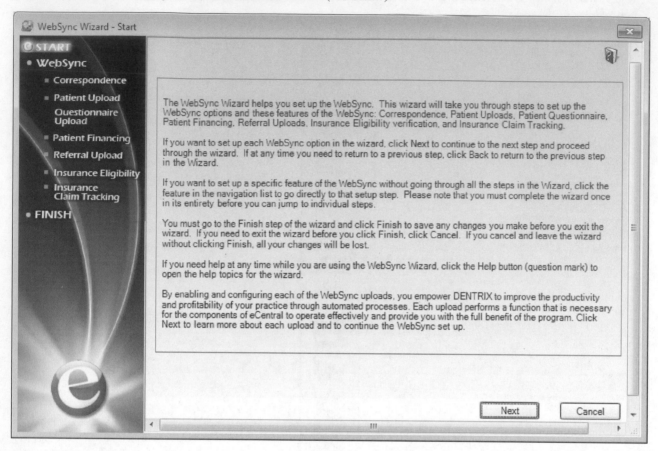

5. Mark **Do Not Run WebSync Automatically** in the Schedule WebSync section of the **WebSync** screen (see below). Do not change the rest of the settings on the screen.

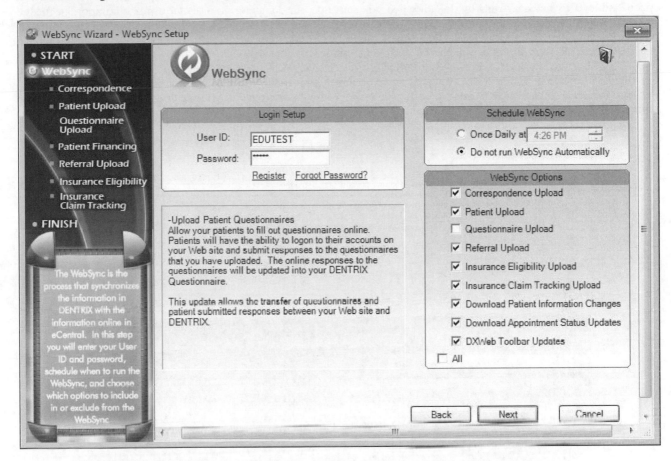

6. Click **Next** on each subsequent screen until you get to the end of the Wizard.

7. Click **Finish** to close the WebSync Wizard.

8. Click the small "X" in the bottom right corner of the DXWeb Toolbar to close it.

NOTE: WebSync is set to start up each time you restart your computer and to run in the background while you work. This is beneficial for offices because they need to use the WebSync functionality throughout the day. Since you do not need to use WebSync, you can remove it from your Windows Startup folder and prevent it from starting up and running.

*To remove WebSync from your Startup folder, click the Windows **Start** button and click **All Programs**. Right-click the folder called **Startup** and click **Open All Users**. In the folder that opens, right-click the **eSync** icon and click **Delete**. Click **Yes** to the message that appears. WebSync will be deleted from the Windows Startup tasks and will not open on your computer again.*

Disabling the Practice Assistant Task Manager

The Practice Assistant Task Manager is used by the Dentrix Practice Assistant to schedule reports to be generated at a specific time. This manager runs by default when you start up your computer. In a dental office it's important for the task manager to be running so that the correct reports are generated at the scheduled time. However, because you will not be scheduling reports to run automatically with the Dentrix Learning Edition, you will not need to run the Practice Assistant Task Manager. Instead, you should disable the manager.

You will not see any messages from the Practice Assistant Task Manager until you shut down your computer. The Practice Assistant Task Manager does not shut down automatically, and it will display a warning message when you try to shut down the computer. After you dismiss that message, while the computer is shutting down, you may see a message telling you that a program is running and you have to force it to close, and it will list the Practice Assistant Task Manager.

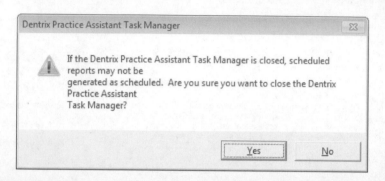

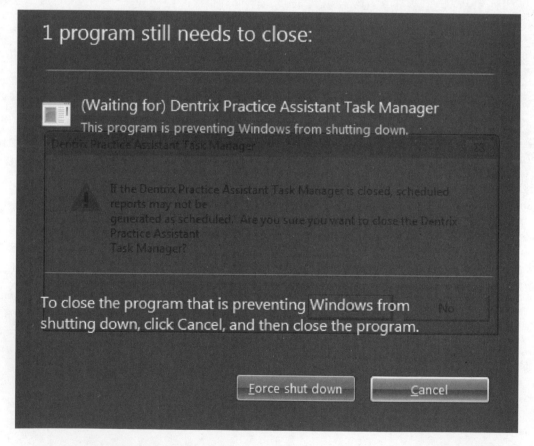

NOTE: It's important to disable the Practice Assistant Task Manager so you don't receive warning messages about the Practice Assistant when you shut down your computer.

Follow the steps below to disable the **Practice Assistant Task Manager**:

1. Locate the **Practice Assistant Task Manager** icon in the Windows Notification Area. If the icon appears in the Notification Area, skip to step 2. If the icon does not appear in the Notification Area, follow steps a and b.

   a. Click the Windows **Start** button, select **All Programs**, and select **Startup** from the menu.

   b. Select **PA Manager** from the Startup menu. The **Practice Assistant Task Manager** icon appears in the Notification Area (see below.)

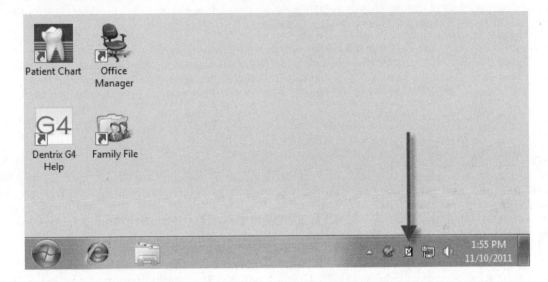

2. Double-click the **Practice Assistant Task Manager** icon. The **Practice Assistant Task Manager** dialog box appears (see below).

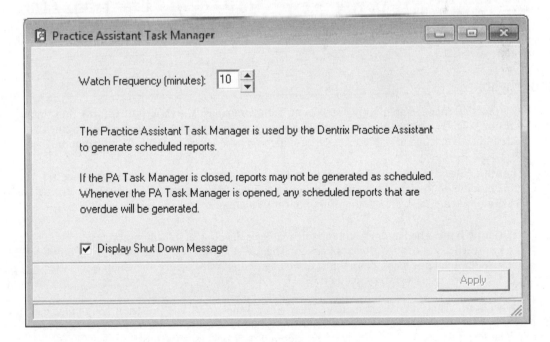

3. Un-check the **Display Shut Down Message** option. This will prevent you from receiving a warning message when you shut down your computer.

4. Click the close button (the "X") in the top right corner of the dialog box to close it.

NOTE: The Apply button in the dialog box may be grayed out. You do not need to click Apply in order to save the changes; you just need to check the option and close the dialog box.

5. Once you have disabled the shutdown message, right-click the **Practice Assistant Task Manager** icon in the Notification Area and click **Close Practice Assistant Manager**.

NOTE: The Practice Assistant Task Manager is set to start up each time you restart your computer. You will not see the messages like those shown above at shutdown if you have followed the steps above, but you may still see a message telling you that the program is still running in the background. If you do not want to see that message, you can remove the Practice Assistant Task Manager from your Startup folder.

*To remove the Practice Assistant Task Manager from your Startup folder, click the Windows **Start** button and click **All Programs**. Right-click the folder called **Startup** and click **Open All Users**. In the folder that opens, right-click the **Practice Assistant Task Manager** icon and click **Delete**. Click **Yes** to the message that appears. The Practice Assistant Task Manager will be deleted from the Windows Startup tasks and will not open on your computer again.*

Congratulations! You have installed your copy of the Dentrix Learning Edition. If you need help, you can use any of the resources listed below.

On-Demand Training

Additional information, including on-demand software tutorials, can be found on the On-Demand Training web page. The tutorials explain fundamental concepts and guide you through hands-on practice exercises. You can even check your understanding with simple quizzes.

To access on-demand training, from any Dentrix module, click **Help > On-Demand Training**. If you have an Internet connection, the On-Demand Training web page opens.

Help Files

To access the Help files, open any module and click **Help > Contents**. The Dentrix Help window appears. In the Help, you can use the navigation tree on the Contents tab to find a feature in a specific module. Or you can type key words in the field on the Search tab to get a list of Help topics.

User's Guide

The Dentrix G4 User's Guide is provided in electronic format on the Dentrix Learning Edition DVD and is saved on the Windows Desktop when you install the Learning Edition. With electronic documentation, you can quickly search for the information you need.

DENTRIX OVERVIEW

As a clinical and practice management software system, Dentrix manages a variety of information, including patient demographics, clinical details, and production analysis. To simplify the process of entering and finding data, the Dentrix software is divided into five separate modules, each of which manages specific types of information.

 Family File: The Family File module manages patient demographic and insurance information. From this module you will keep track of a patient's name, address, employer, insurance information, notes, and continuing care, as well as other important information.

 Patient Chart: The Patient Chart module manages the clinical information for patients. The Patient Chart is a powerful, yet easy-to-use, application. The Chart allows you to post existing, completed, and recommended procedures using common textbook symbols. Additionally, the Chart helps users keep extensive and detailed notes regarding patient care.

Several submodules of the Chart help users manage other clinical functions. The Presenter is a unique case presentation program that displays the treatment plan costs in terms of primary and secondary insurance portions and the estimated patient portion. The Perio Chart is an unparalleled periodontal data maintenance tool.

Ledger: Patient accounts are managed in the Ledger. Because Dentrix is a seamlessly integrated system, procedures completed in the Patient Chart are automatically posted in the Ledger. All financial transactions are recorded in the Ledger, including charges, payments, and adjustments. The Ledger provides information concerning patient portion versus insurance portion, deductibles owed, and payment arrangements.

 Office Manager: The Office Manager offers useful, customizable reports including day sheets, aging reports, financial reports, patient lists, reference reports, and more.

Additionally, the Office Manager integrates with Microsoft Word to create effective, professional-looking letters that are available at the click of a mouse. These letters include welcome letters, congratulatory letters, thank you letters, and a variety of appointment and continuing care (recall) reminders, progress reports, and collection notices. The Office Manager contains a set of utilities and commands that make customizing Dentrix easy.

 Appointment Book: Managing appointments has never been easier than with the Dentrix Appointment Book. The Appointment Book offers all the functionality of the Appointment List in a user-friendly graphical interface. The Appointment Book offers goal-oriented scheduling with the flexibility to make one-time changes.

The Appointment Book's convenient toolbars and Flip Tabs make navigating through the Appointment Book, searching for open times, and organizing appointments simple and quick. With the click of a button, the Appointment Book allows you to schedule appointments, record broken appointments, print route slips, and dial a patient's phone number directly from the computer. And like the standard Dentrix modules, the Appointment Book provides access to other Dentrix modules from the toolbar.

Important Buttons to Know

 Patient Chart: This button appears on every major toolbar throughout Dentrix except within the Patient Chart module. Click this button to open and display the current patient's chart.

 Family File: This button appears on every major toolbar throughout Dentrix except within the Family File. Click this button to open and display the current patient's family file.

 Ledger: This button appears on every major toolbar throughout Dentrix except within the Ledger. Click this button to open and display the current patient's ledger.

 Appointments: This button appears on every major toolbar throughout Dentrix except within the Appointment Book or Appointment List. Click this button to open the Appointment Book (if installed) or the Appointment List to the current date (the current system date).

 Office Manager: This button appears on every major toolbar throughout Dentrix except within the Office Manager. Click this button to open the Office Manager.

 Select Patient: This button appears on every major toolbar throughout Dentrix except within the Office Manager and the Appointment Book. Click this button to select a patient from the patient database.

 Quick Letters: This button appears on every major toolbar throughout Dentrix except within the Office Manager. Click this button to print prewritten letters concerning a patient's account or clinical diagnosis and treatment plan.

 Continuing Care (Recall): This button appears on every major toolbar throughout Dentrix except within the Office Manager. Click this button to view recall appointments assigned to a patient and track whether or not an appointment has been made.

 Office Journal: This button appears on every major toolbar throughout Dentrix except within the Office Journal. The Office Journal acts as a contact manager for your dental office. All correspondence and contacts made with patients can be tracked and recorded by clicking the Office Journal button.

xxxv

Questionnaires: This button appears on every major toolbar throughout Dentrix except within the Office Manager. Click this button to open the Questionnaires module from which you can view questionnaires, enter questionnaire responses, sign questionnaires, and update the Family File with information provided through questionnaire responses. The Questionnaires button looks like a blank form when the selected patient does not have any questionnaire responses attached. The Questionnaires button looks like a form with a red check mark when the patient has questionnaire responses attached.

 Prescriptions: This button appears on every major toolbar throughout Dentrix except within the Office Manager. Click this button to open a window from which prescriptions can be printed and a notation that a drug has been prescribed can be made.

 Medical Alerts: This button appears on the Family File, Patient Chart, and Presenter toolbars. The button is red when a patient has a health condition requiring attention. Click this button to open a list of a patient's medical alerts. Medical alerts can be added, edited, or deleted from this list.

 Patient Picture: This button appears on all modules except within the Ledger and Office Manager. Click this button to open a digital photograph of the selected patient. If no picture is assigned to the patient, the icon will be a graphic of a framed photo. If a picture is assigned to the patient, the icon will be a miniature of that picture.

 Patient Alerts: This button appears on every major toolbar throughout Dentrix except within the Office Manager. Click this button to add or edit Patient Alerts for the selected patient.

 Document Center: This button appears on every major toolbar throughout Dentrix except within the Document Center. Click this button to open the Document Center window in which documents can be viewed, edited, and attached to patients, providers, employers, referrals, and insurance carriers. The Document Center icon looks like a closed filing cabinet if the selected patient does not have documents attached in the Document Center module. The Document Center icon looks like a filing cabinet with paper in the open drawer if the selected patient has documents attached in the Document Center module.

 Patient Referrals: This button appears on every major toolbar throughout Dentrix except within the Office Manager. Click this button to open a window in which patient referral information can be viewed, added, or edited.

 Treatment Planner: This button appears only in the Patient Chart module. Click this button to create new treatment plan cases, sign treatment consent forms, and view treatment case totals. The Treatment Planner button appears green when a treatment plan is saved for the selected patient.

 Presenter: This button appears only in the Patient Chart module. Click this button to present treatment case information and view patient education.

 Perio: This button appears only in the Patient Chart module. Click this button to chart perio scores, enter oral health data, and compare current oral health with previous exams. The Perio button has a blue background when a perio exam has been saved for the selected patient.

 Guru: This button appears only in the Patient Chart module. Click this button to launch Guru Limited Edition or Henry Schein Guru (if you have the full version installed), where you can view patient education topics, create patient education playlists, and create custom patient education topics.

USER SUPPORT

For technical support regarding the **installation** of Dentrix Learning Edition, first refer to the *Dentrix G4 User's Guide* found on the DVD-ROM. Further **installation support** is available by contacting Dentrix directly via phone at 1-800-DENTRIX (336-8749) or via email at support@dentrix.com. Further support information and options can be accessed at www.dentrix.com/support/contact-us.aspx. Questions about the exercises or functionality of the program should be directed to your instructor. All Dentrix content within this section courtesy Henry Schein Practice Solutions, American Fork, Utah.

1.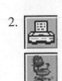

Icon _____ Type of Information _____

2.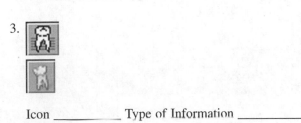

Icon _____ Type of Information _____

3.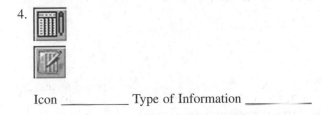

Icon _____ Type of Information _____

4.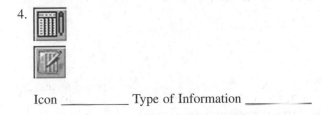

Icon _____ Type of Information _____

a. Manages employee information

b. Manages the clinical information of the patient

c. Manages patient demographic and insurance information

d. Manages the patient's appointment information

e. Generates reports, creates patient letters, and sends insurance claims

f. Provides information about the patient's financial transactions

7

Provider and Staff Setup

To view the practice information, in the Office Manager, select **Maintenance—Practice Setup—Practice Resource Setup.** The Practice Resource Setup dialogue box appears.

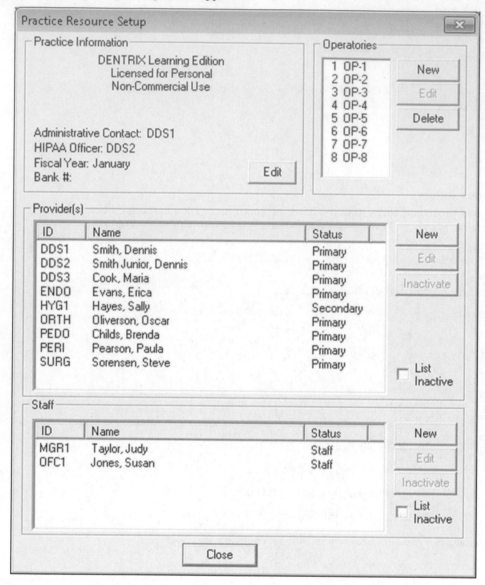

Answer the following questions with the information located in the **Practice Resource Setup** dialogue box:

1. Who is the Administrative Contact (name)?

2. What dental specialty does Dr. Brenda Childs practice?

3. If a patient needed to be scheduled for a root canal what provider would you select?

4. Who is the office manager?

Click **Close.**

Please note: With the commercial edition of Dentrix, you will have the ability to set up and edit practice information, providers, and staff members.

Operatory Setup

To add a new operatory:

1. In the Office Manager, select **Maintenance—Practice Setup—Practice Resource Setup**. The Practice Resource Setup dialogue box appears (see above).

2. In the Operatories group box, click **New.**

3. Enter an ID for the operatory in the **ID** field (enter the first four letters of your name). This information will appear as an operatory in the appointment book.

4. Enter a description (use your name).

5. Click **Close.**

Procedure Codes Setup

You can set up new procedure codes to fit the needs of your office. The Learning Edition does not include the standard CDT codes. Because of copyright reasons, they have been replaced with non-ADA codes.

1. In the Office Manager, select **Maintenance—Practice Setup—Procedure Code Setup.** The Procedure Code Setup dialogue box appears.

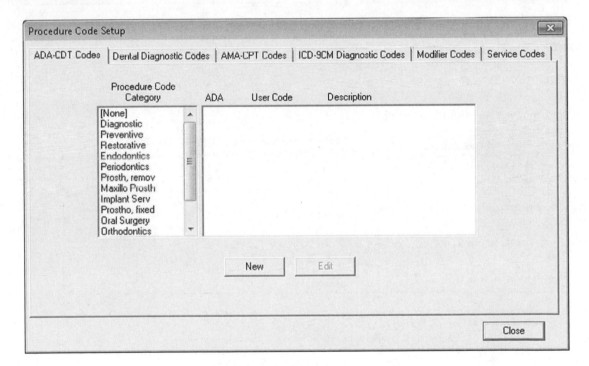

Chapter **1 Orientation to the Dental Profession**

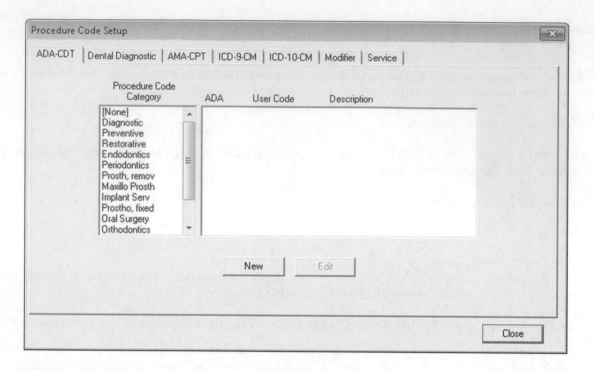

2. Click the **ADA-CDT Codes** tab Preventative and scroll through the Procedure Code Categories until you locate **X2397.**

3. Click **Edit.**

Answer the following questions:

1. What is the name of the dialogue box?

2. What is the *Description?*

3. What is the fee charged BC/BS?

4. Edit the fee for Aetna to $54.00.

Click **Save** and **Close.**

Fee Schedule Setup

The Automatic Fee Schedule Changes utility allows you to change an entire fee schedule rather than changing one fee at a time. To use the Automatic Fee Schedule Changes utility

1. In the Office Manager, select **Maintenance—Practice Setup—Auto Fee Schedule Changes.** The Automatic Fee Schedule Changes dialogue box appears:

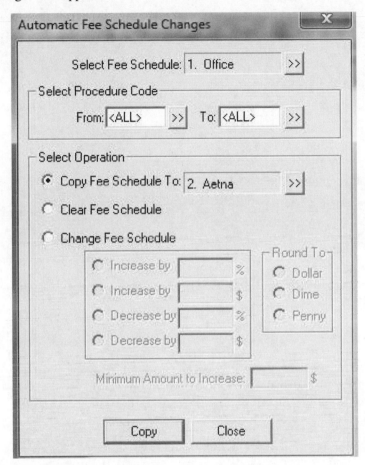

Note: The default should be **Select Fee Schedule** 1. Office and **Select Procedure Code**, from <All> to <All> Please change if necessary.

2. In *Select Operation,* click—**Change Fee Schedule.**

3. Increase the fees by 8%.

4. Click—**Change.**

5. Scroll to procedure code **X1772** and click on it to select.

   Answer the following questions:

   ■ What was the *Fee #1 Office?*

   ■ What is the new fee?

6. Click **Edit.**

7. Change the fee to $130.00.

8. Click to save **(check mark).**

9. Click **Accept.**

10. Click **Close.**

To review all the setup features in detail refer to the Dentrix *User's Guide.*

2 Dental Basics

LEARNING OBJECTIVES

1. List and describe the different areas of a dental office.
2. Identify the basic structures of the face and oral cavity, including the basic anatomical structures and tissues of the teeth.
3. Distinguish between different tooth-numbering systems.
4. Interpret dental-charting symbols.
5. Categorize basic dental procedures.
6. List basic chairside dental assisting duties and identify Occupational Safety and Health Administration (OSHA) and state regulations.

INTRODUCTION

The administrative dental assistant has a unique opportunity to communicate in several "languages." You will be a translator between the dental community and the patient. As part of your job, you will represent the dentist when you communicate with dental professionals, dental insurance companies, patients, vendors, and fellow team members. Patients are often unwilling or unable to ask the dentist questions directly, so they will turn to the assistants for clarification. To be an effective communicator, you must first understand the language of dentistry.

EXERCISES

1. Identify the different areas of the dental practice.

   a. _____ The first area to be viewed by the patient.

   b. _____ Area used by administrative dental assistants to perform daily business tasks.

   c. _____ A private area used to discuss confidential information with a patient.

   d. _____ Area where duties pertaining to the fiscal operation of the dental practice take place.

   e. _____ Area where patients are treated by the dentist, dental hygienist, and dental assistant.

   f. _____ Consists of a contaminated area and a clean area.

   g. _____ Dental x-rays are taken in this area.

   h. _____ Dental radiographic film is processed in this area.

   A. Sterilization area

   B. Clinical area

   C. Reception area

   D. Business office

   E. Nonclinical areas

   F. Staff room

   G. Darkroom

   H. Treatment rooms

   I. Consultation area

   J. Radiology room

   K. Storage area

2. Label the following diagram:

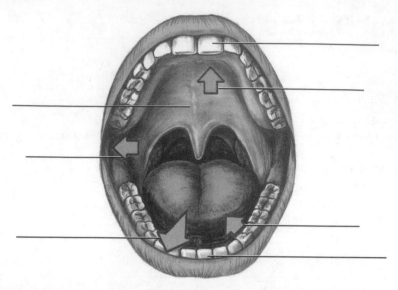

(From Fehrenbach MJ, Herring SW: *Illustrated anatomy of the head and neck,* ed 3, St. Louis, 2007, Saunders.)

3. Label the following diagram:

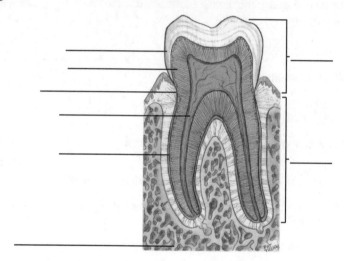

(From Bath-Balogh M, Fehrenbach MF: *Illustrated dental embryology, histology, and anatomy,* ed 3, St. Louis, 2011, Saunders.)

Using the patient chart below, complete the following tasks:

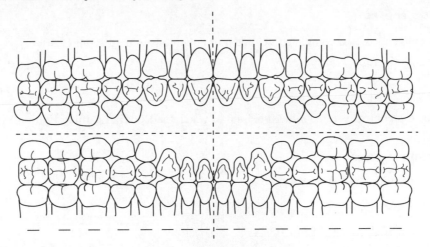

(From Bird DL, Robinson DS: *Modern dental assisting,* ed 10, St. Louis, 2012, Saunders.)

4. Correctly number the teeth on the chart (space provided on the chart above the maxillary arch and below the mandibular arch) using the Universal/National Numbering System.

5. Correctly chart the following conditions using the symbols described in Chapter 2 (use red and blue or black pencil):

   a. Maxillary right third molar, impacted

   b. Maxillary right second molar, MO restoration

   c. Maxillary right second premolar, MOD caries

   d. Maxillary right central, bonded veneer

   e. Maxillary left central, bonded veneer

   f. Maxillary left first molar, DO restoration

   g. Maxillary left third molar, missing

   h. Mandibular left third molar, missing

   i. Mandibular left first molar, full gold crown

   j. Mandibular left cuspid, periapical abscess

   k. Mandibular right lateral, mesial composite

   l. Mandibular right second premolar, occlusal caries

   m. Mandibular right first molar, completed endodontic treatment, post and core, PFM

   n. Mandibular right third molar, needs to be extracted

Dentrix Learning Objectives

■ Post existing, recommended, and completed treatment or conditions in the Patient Chart.

■ Print a Patient Chart.

Getting Started

Before you begin this assignment you may find it helpful to watch the Dentrix Learning Edition Videos and review the Dentrix User's Guide:

Dentrix Learning Edition Video

http://www.dentrix.com/le/on-demand-training

Patient Chart

■ Viewing and Navigating the Patient Chart

■ Quiz

■ Customizing the Patient Chart

■ Quiz

■ Charting and Editing Treatment

■ Quiz

Dentrix User's Guide

Chapter 4: Patient Chart

■ The Patient Chart Window

■ Entering Treatment

■ Editing Treatment

■ Chart Customization

■ Printing the Patient Chart

■ Chart Shortcuts and Tips

Dentrix Practice

Posting treatment to the patient chart

Keeping an electronic record of your patient's treatment is the primary way treatment is charted. In most dental offices the clinical dental assistant completes charting during the examination and records procedures after each dental visit. To help expand your skills the following is a brief introduction to electronic dental charting.

Study the Patient Chart Window in the Dentrix User's Guide

Be able to locate:

■ Procedure Codes

■ Procedure Buttons

■ Status Buttons (including drop down lists)

■ Progress Notes

You can select the procedure you would like to post in one of three ways

■ Selecting *Procedure buttons*

■ Selecting procedure codes from the *Procedure Codes panel* or

- Manually enter the procedure code into *Procedure Code Listing field*.

    Status Buttons Definitions

- **Existing Other (EO)** is for work completed by another provider or practice.

- **Existing (Ex)** is for work done by the current provider, but is just now being entered into the Patient Chart

- **Treatment Plan (Tx)** is for treatment–planned procedures.

- **Completed (?)** is for completed procedures.

Tip: No matter what method you use to post the procedure you must have a procedure code listed in the Procedure Code Listing field, this will occur when you select a procedure from the Procedure Codes panel and click the **Post** button; when you select a button from the **Procedure Buttons;** or manually enter the code into the **Procedure Code Listing** field. You will not select a tooth if you are entering a procedure that does not require a tooth number such as radiographs, or examinations.

Posting Procedures in the Dentrix Patient Chart

1. In the Patient Chart module, select a patient. Click the **Select Patient** button and type in the first few letters of the patient's last name. For this exercise your patient will be Michelle Keller. You will be selecting procedure codes from the Procedure Codes panel.

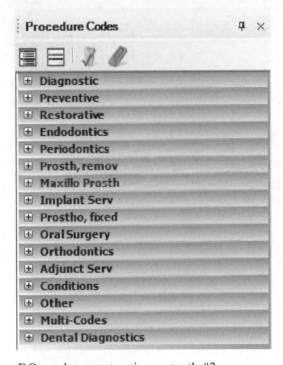

You will be charting an existing DO amalgam restoration on tooth #2.

2. Select **tooth #2** in the Graphic Chart.

3. Select the procedure category from the Procedure Code panel (such as Diagnostic, Preventive, Restorative, and son on.) Click **Restorative**. The list will expand with procedure codes and a description.

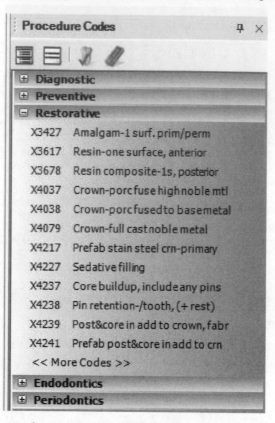

Tip: If the code is not listed you may have to expand the list; scroll to the end of the list and click ≪**more codes**≫

4. Select the desired procedure. You will need to expand the list scroll to the end and click ≪**more codes**≫ Select **X3437 Amalgam-2-surf. Prim/perm**

5. Click the **Post** Button. (Check and make sure the code is listed in the Procedure Code field.)

6. Click the desired Status button: Click **Existing (Ex).** The Select Surface dialog box appears.

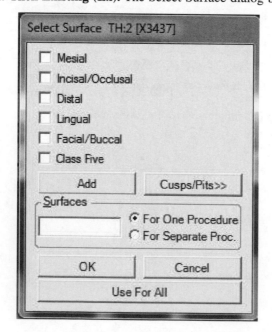

7. Check the desired surfaces, **Distal and Occlusal**.

8. Click **OK**.

If everything was done correctly you should see that tooth #2 on the Graphic Chart now illustrates a DO restoration in blue and the tooth is listed in the Progress Notes with a status of E.

Tip: To delete a procedure highlight the desired procedure in the Progress Notes block and click the Delete Control button in the Progress Notes toolbar (or right click and select Delete.)

Entering Treatment for Multiple Teeth

Occasionally you may have the same procedure to enter for multiple teeth. This can be done by selecting all of the teeth on the Graphic Chart prior to entering the procedure code.

For this exercise you are going to enter that all four 3rd molars have been extracted (fully erupted) by a previous dentist.

1. Select teeth numbers **1, 16, 17, and 32** in the Graphic Chart.

2. Click **Oral Surgery** in the Procedure Code panel.

3. Select procedure code **X8057 Extraction Surgical/erupt. Tooth**

4. Click **Post** (Did the procedure code appear in the Procedure Code List field?)

5. Select Status. Click **Existing Other (EO)**

Did the teeth disappear from the Graphic Chart? And is there a notation in the Progress Chart with a status of EO? If you answered YES, congratulations, if not go back and try again.

Entering Treatment that Requires Quadrant(s)

If you select a procedure that requires quadrants such as periodontal scaling, the Learning Edition prompts you to select the applicable quadrants. For this exercise you are going to enter planned treatment for four quadrants fo periodontal sclaing.

1. Select the procedure code from the Procedure Code panel. Click **Periodontics**.

2. Select the procedure code. **X5629 Perio Scaling & root pln 1-3 quad.**

3. Click **Post**.

4. Select Status button. Click **Tx**. The Select Quadrant box appears.

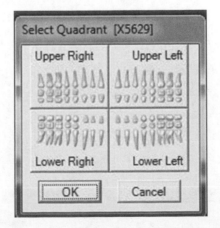

5. Select the quadrants. Click **Upper Right, Lower Right, Upper Left, Lower Left**

6. Click **OK**

Note: For this procedure you will not see anything post to the Graphic Chart, but you will see the procedures listed in the Progress Notes.

On your own post the following treatment to Michelle's chart.

1. Treatment plan a root canal (Endodontics X4617), post & core (Restorative, X4241) and porcelain fused to high noble crown (Restorative, X4037) for tooth number 30.

   Tip: You can select all procedures in the Procedure Code panel before clicking the Post button.

2. Completed MOD composite for tooth number 29

3. Existing Distal composites to teeth numbers 8 & 9

Printing a Patient Chart

If you want to give your patient a copy of their chart, you can print the Patient Chart.

To print the Patient Chart:

1. In the Patient Chart for your patient Michelle Keller, click the **Print Patient Chart** button (on the Progress Notes toolbar). The Print Patient Chart dialog box appears.

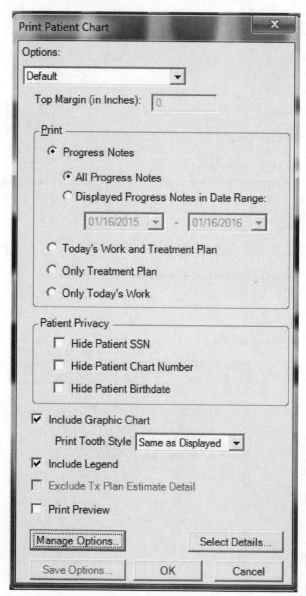

"You" technique: _____

_____

_____

_____

Organization: _____

_____

_____

_____

2. Compose one or two sentences that are examples of

Tone: _____

_____

_____

_____

Outlook: _____

_____

_____

_____

"You" technique: _____

_____

_____

_____

3. Match each of the following statements with the correct title:

a. _____ Address of the party receiving the letter.

b. _____ Alert the reader that there is more to the letter.

c. _____ Describes what the next step or expected outcome will be.

d. _____ Draws attention to the person you wish to read the letter.

e. _____ Draws attention to the subject of the correspondence.

f. _____ Final closing of the letter and is a courtesy.

g. _____ First paragraph and states the reason you are writing.

h. _____ Gives details of the points that you stated in the introduction.

i. _____ Greeting.

j. _____ Identifies the dental practice that is sending the letter.

k. _____ Identifies the writer of the letter.

l. _____ Is used when the sender of the letter is representing the company.

m. _____ The date the letter was written.

n. _____ Includes three sections.

o. _____ Used to identify the sender and the typist of the letter.

p. _____ Used to notify the reader that a copy of the document is being forwarded to another party.

A. Subject line

B. Signer's identification

C. Salutation

D. Reference initials

E. Main body

F. Line spacing

G. Letterhead

H. Introduction

I. Inside address

J. Enclosure reminder

K. Date line

L. Copy notation

M. Complimentary closing

N. Company signature

O. Closing

P. Body of the letter

Q. Attention lines

4. All letter sections begin at the left margin, and proper spacing is applied between sections.

a. Full-Blocked

b. Blocked

c. Semi-Blocked

d. Square-Blocked

e. Simplified or AMS

5. Date line is on the same line as the first line of the inside address and is right justified. Reference initials and enclosure reminders are typed on the same line as the signer's identification and are right justified.

a. Full-Blocked

b. Blocked

c. Semi-Blocked

d. Square-Blocked

e. Simplified or AMS

6. Same as blocked with one change; paragraphs are indented five spaces.

   a. Full-Blocked

   b. Blocked

   c. Semi-Blocked

   d. Square-Blocked

   e. Simplified or AMS

7. Margins are the same as full-blocked, with the exception of date line, complimentary close, company signature, and writer's identification.

   a. Full-Blocked

   b. Blocked

   c. Semi-Blocked

   d. Square-Blocked

   e. Simplified or AMS

8. Style is fast and efficient.

   a. Full-Blocked

   b. Blocked

   c. Semi-Blocked

   d. Square-Blocked

   e. Simplified or AMS

As the administrative dental assistant it is your responsibility to process outgoing mail. In the following scenarios, identify the type of mail service you would select.

9. You have just completed the quarterly newsletter (350 newsletters). The newsletters are bundled according to the specifications of the postal service.

   What type of postage has been used? _____

10. At the end of the day you have completed several insurance claims for the same carrier. It is important the claims arrive in the next 2 days.

    What service of the USPS will you use? _____

    What is the current rate for this type of service? _____

11. Joel Curren has an appointment tomorrow at 4:30 PM with an oral surgeon. You have been asked by Dr. Edwards to send a referral letter and x-rays.

    What type of service will you use to ensure the information is received in time for his appointment?

    _____

29

12. Dr. Bradley has just seen an emergency patient of Dr. Coffee's and has prepared a report. The patient is due back in Dr. Coffee's office this afternoon for a follow-up appointment.

What information do you need to send, and how will you ensure that it will arrive on time and be HIPAA compliant?

ACTIVITY EXERCISE

13. Complete the following tasks using the information below:

    - Write a referral letter. (Create letterhead using the examples in textbook Chapter 4 for Dr. Edwards.)

    - Use word processing software.

    - Select a letter style of your choice.

    - Use your initials in the reference initials.

    - Address an envelope. (Use a real envelope or draw a business envelope.)

Joel is being referred to Donald Payne, DDS, 23454 Tenth Street, Suite 234, Canyon View, California 91786, Attention Joan. The referral is for the extraction of teeth numbers 1, 16, 17, and 32. Joel is 18 years old and will be leaving for college in 3 weeks.

WHAT WOULD YOU DO?

You have been asked to create a guideline for the dental office on sending e-mail messages. In your guideline you need to cover the type of messages that should be sent via e-mail, examples of good subject lines, and how to get the response you want. Also, identify what information can be sent over an unsecured e-mail server and what types of messages need to be secure.

Hint: Do an Internet search on "how to write an effective e-mail."

5 Patient Relations

LEARNING OBJECTIVES

1. Compare and contrast the humanistic theory according to Maslow and Rogers. Relate the theory to patient relations.
2. List the different stages that present a positive image for the dental practice.
3. Describe the elements of a positive image and give examples.
4. Demonstrate different problem-solving techniques.
5. Examine different methods of providing outstanding customer service. Discuss team strategies and personal strategies for providing exceptional patient care.

INTRODUCTION

Patient relations involve empathy, understanding, concern, and warmth for each patient. These emotions can be demonstrated in the way we communicate with patients, in the type of service we provide, in how members of the dental healthcare team relate to each other, and in how problems are solved. Every aspect of the dental practice should be conducted with the understanding that the patient is "number one."

EXERCISES

1. Match the following statements with the corresponding stage:

   a. _____ Advertisement

   b. _____ Amount of information given

   c. _____ Answers to questions match individual needs

   d. _____ Appearance of the reception area

   e. _____ Attitude and professionalism meet expectations

   f. _____ Communication skills of the staff and dentist

   g. _____ Financial arrangements meet needs

   h. _____ How the telephone is answered

   i. _____ Name of dental practice

   j. _____ Office is easy to find

   k. _____ Talking with friends

   l. _____ Time spent waiting

   A. Investigation Stage

   B. Initial Contact Stage

   C. Confirmation of Initial Impression Stage

   D. Final Decision Stage

2. What can be done to ensure that patients' expectations are being met? List the eight points (summarize).

_____

_____

_____

_____

_____

_____

_____

_____

_____

_____

In the following scenario, the administrative dental assistant is faced with a typical daily problem. Michele Austin is a 32-year-old patient who has been scheduled three different times for completion of a root canal. Each time when you call and confirm the appointment, she finds some reason to postpone it. She has told you that her schedule at work is very busy and she cannot leave, that her daughter has a dance recital, and that she has to make final arrangements for the family dinner party. You have just called her for the fourth time, and this time, she informs you that she will be leaving on vacation next week and wants to wait until she gets back.

3. What steps would you take to identify the problem? (With information given in the scenario, use your imagination and list the problem or problems.)

_____

_____

_____

_____

_____

_____

_____

4. Based on your selected problem, what steps will you take to solve this problem? Is there more than one way to solve the problem?

_____

_____

_____

_____

_____

5. Can the problem be prevented in the future? If so, how?

_____

_____

_____

_____

6. Identify strategies that can be used by the dental healthcare team to provide outstanding customer (patient) service.

_____

_____

_____

_____

_____

_____

_____

_____

7. Based on your personal experiences, which is the most important of these strategies (from Question 6), and why?

_____

_____

_____

_____

_____

_____

_____

WHAT WOULD YOU DO?

You have been asked to work with a small team of colleagues (clinical assistant, dental hygienist, and associate dentist) to explore the development of a practice website. The practice is opening a new location, and the primary purpose of the site is to introduce the dental practice to the community. You have been asked to give your opinion on the following:

1. What do you think should be included on the website?

2. What are the legal and ethical advertising guidelines the dental practice needs to follow?

3. Provide examples of websites that meet your criteria and explain why.

Hint: Do an Internet search for "dental websites" and search the American Dental Association (ADA) website for advertising information.

6 Dental Healthcare Team Communications

LEARNING OBJECTIVES

1. Discuss the purpose of a dental practice procedural manual and identify the different elements of the manual.
2. Categorize the various channels of organizational communication and identify the types of communication that are used in each channel.
3. Identify and discuss barriers to organizational communications.
4. Describe different types of organizational conflict and select the appropriate style for resolution.
5. Explain the purpose of staff meetings.

INTRODUCTION

A team can be described as a group of two or more persons who work toward a common goal. Similar to those on a sports team, all members must understand and practice established rules and have a common goal. An effective healthcare team requires a shared philosophy, excellent communication skills, the desire to grow and change, and the ability to be flexible while providing quality care for all patients.

EXERCISES

1. List the main elements of a procedural manual.

   _____

   _____

   _____

   _____

   _____

2. Identify the four channels of organizational communication, and give two examples for each channel.

   _____

   _____

   _____

   _____

   _____

Identify the type of barrier to organizational communication that may result in the following scenarios:

3. Kim tells the office manager about a new idea she has that will improve the insurance billing process. The office

   manager decides not to tell the dentist about the idea. Classify the barrier. _____

4. Julie has a very full schedule as the receptionist. Kim, the insurance clerk, calls in sick and tells Julie that the daily insurance claims must be processed by the end of the day and asks if she will take on the responsibility of completing the task. Classify the barrier. _____

5. Kim is told that she will not get paid for her sick day because she did not report the absence correctly. Kim questions the ruling because it is the first time she has been informed that there is a reporting policy. Classify the barrier.

_____

6. Julie is excited about a new seminar that is being offered. She tries to explain the seminar to the dentist on his way out of the office to meet with the accountant. She is disappointed when he does not share in her excitement. Classify the barrier. _____

7. Organizational conflict can be described as _____ (conflict within the organization) and _____ (conflict between two or more organizations).

8. Define the four types of intraorganizational conflict.
   ■ Intrapersonal Conflict:

   _____

   _____

   _____

   ■ Interpersonal Conflict:

   _____

   _____

   _____

   ■ Intragroup Conflict:

   _____

   _____

   _____

   ■ Intergroup Conflict:

   _____

   _____

   _____

9. Identify and define the five conflict-handling styles, according to Rahim and Bonoma.

_____

_____

_____

_____

_____

What style of conflict resolution would be appropriate for the following problems (support your answer)?

10. Problem: A new computer system is needed.

_____

_____

_____

_____

11. Problem: You don't like the color of the new uniform, and everyone else thinks it is great. (You will have to wear this color only once a week.)

_____

_____

_____

_____

12. Problem: Dr. Edwards takes 2 weeks off during the summer and closes her office. Her staff cannot agree on a vacation schedule for all of them; therefore, Dr. Edwards sets the date and does not offer any options.

_____

_____

_____

_____

13. Problem: Julie and Kim both want to leave early to get ready for the long weekend. One person will have to stay until 6 PM to check out the last patient. Julie agrees to stay only if Kim will open for her on Tuesday morning.

_____

_____

_____

_____

14. State the purpose of a staff meeting at the beginning of each day.

_____

_____

_____

_____

DENTAL PRACTICE PROCEDURAL MANUAL PROJECT (OPTIONAL)

The dental practice procedural manual is a detailed manual that is used as a form of written communication. The objective of the manual is to provide a reference for all team members. This resource provides each team member with specific details on practice goals, personnel procedures, business office procedures, and clinical procedures. The manual should be developed as a team project, with each team member contributing in his or her specific area of expertise. As procedures change, it is the team members' responsibility to update the manual. To be effective, the manual must be updated at regular intervals and all team members must be given updated manuals.

The key to developing a good procedural manual is to include as much information as possible without making the manual cumbersome. The idea is for the manual to be a resource for all team members. It will not be used on a daily basis by experienced team members but it will be used to help train new team members and will serve as a guide for substitute team members or, when necessary, for a team member who fills in for another. The purposes of the manual are to provide written documentation of and to eliminate inconsistency in policies. Such inconsistencies are a common cause of conflict among members of the dental healthcare team.

Project Overview

During this project, which spans the full textbook, your team will do research, have discussions, and come to consensus about the information you will include in your procedural manual. The majority of the information your team will need will be in the textbook and created during Career Ready Practices exercises at the end of each chapter. In addition you will need to do some research to find additional information.

How to approach the project:

1. Work as a team (although the project is designed as a team activity, it can be completed by individuals).

2. Name your dental practice.

3. Identify the roles and responsibilities of each team member. Develop a timeline to complete the project. How will the work be divided? How will the team discuss key issues? How will you resolve conflict?

4. Build upon previous activities presented in the text, for example, Career Ready Practices exercises, and What Would You Do scenarios.

5. Review procedural manuals from dental practices for ideas. You can obtain some online or ask a local dental practice for a copy of their manual. Remember these are only samples; some may be very good, while others may be outdated or missing information.

6. Your manual will have key components but will not have all the information that should be included in a comprehensive procedural manual; Feel free to expand upon the project and add components and information that is important to your team.

7. Remember you want the manual to be easy to read; for example, information on procedures and job description can be as simple as an overview and a bulleted list.

8. Components of your manual can be completed at the end of the applicable chapter.

9. The finished procedural manual will be word processed and neatly organized. The final project may be used for the team grade.

10. Each team member will keep a journal about his or her role during the project to identify his or her responsibilities, major contributions, and time spent. This journal may be used for an individual grade.

Key Components for the Dental Practice Procedural Manual Project

The following components are a portion of what will be included in a compressive procedural manual. Some of the components are covered in several chapters throughout the textbook and may not be completed at one time, for example, job descriptions; although an overview of the job is given in Chapter 1, the detail will be covered in many other chapters.

Procedural Manual Section	Key Component	Primary Source Chapter
Practice Philosophy	Mission Statement	Chapter 1
General Instructions	Mission Statement for the Manual (team mission)	Chapter 6
	How to Use the Manual	Chapter 6
	Responsibility for Updating and Reviewing	Chapter 6
Personnel Procedures	Hiring	Chapter 18
	Work Schedules	Chapter 10
	Job Descriptions	Several chapters
	Code of Conduct	Chapters 1-6
	Reviews and Evaluations	Chapter 18
	Termination Procedures	Chapter 18
Health Insurance Portability and Accountability Act (HIPAA) Procedures	Identify Who Manages HIPAA Compliance	Chapter 1
	Establish a Plan for Compliance	Chapter 1
	Identify the Components of HIPAA	Chapter 1, covered in several chapters
	Describe the Roles and Responsibilities of Various Members of the Dental Health Care Team	Chapter 1, covered in several chapters
Mandated State and Federal Requirements	Health and Safety	Chapter 12
	Electronic Health Records	Chapter 8
Business Office Procedures	Specific Duties and Job Descriptions (detailed information for each procedure and duty performed in the business office)	Covered in several chapters
	Records Management Protocol (detailed information for each type of record)	Chapter 8
Clinical Area Procedures	Description of the Inventory Procedure	Chapter 12
	Description of the Hazardous Material Program	Chapter 12

Computerized Dental Practice

LEARNING OBJECTIVES

1. Compare the basic and advanced functions of dental practice management software and discuss their application.
2. Explain how to select a dental practice management system and list the functions to consider during the selection process.
3. Discuss the role of the administrative dental assistant in the operation of a computerized dental practice.
4. Identify the daily computer tasks performed by the administrative dental assistant, including the importance of a computer system backup routine.

INTRODUCTION

If you are a digital native (born after 1988), you have grown up in the digital world. The use of computers, cellphones, smartphones, iPods, video games, and other digital tools has always been a part of your world. This is not the case for those of us who are considered immigrants to the digital world. We have performed many tasks in the dental office without the aid of a computer. We have manually maintained clinical records, written in an appointment book, used a one-write (pegboard) system, and manually submitted dental insurance claim forms. Although these practices are still used in many offices, the use of digital technology has become the standard in the majority of dental practices. The fully integrated digital dental practice integrates the functionality of several software systems to seamlessly gather, process, connect, and store digital information, connecting the business office with the clinical practice.

EXERCISES

1. Briefly describe how information is gathered to build a patent's EHR.

40

2. What are the basic business functions of a computerized practice management system?

_____

_____

_____

_____

3. What is the advantage of the additional tools and resources that are provided in more advanced software suites?

_____

_____

_____

_____

4. List the functions you should consider when selecting dental management practice software.

_____

_____

_____

_____

_____

_____

_____

_____

_____

_____

5. In your opinion what are two reasons why a computerized practice management system is important to a dental practice?

_____

_____

Describe the functions of the computerized practice management system that are of use to each of the following members of the dental healthcare team:

6. Accountant: _____

7. Dental hygienist: _____

8. Administrative dental assistant: _____

9. Insurance biller: _____

10. Describe the role of the administrative dental assistant in the operation of a computerized dental practice.

_____

_____

_____

_____

_____

11. What are the advantages of using a computerized system?

_____

_____

_____

_____

_____

_____

12. List the daily procedures performed with the use of computerized dental software.

_____

_____

_____

_____

_____

_____

13. Describe the importance of backing up a computerized dental practice system.

_____

_____

_____

_____

_____

_____

14. Match the following computerized dental practice software terms to their definitions:

a. _____ Appears when additional information is needed   A. Menu Bar

b. _____ Identifies software being used   B. Power Bar

c. _____ Provides information about current screen   C. Status Bar

d. _____ Arranges parts of screens in logical order   D. Status Window

e. _____ Icons and buttons that identify commonly used features E. Tabbed Screen

f. _____ Identifies name of user   F. Title Bar

g. _____ Provides quick access to selected features   G. Toolbar

DENTRIX EXERCISE

Dentrix Learning Objectives
■ Identify key elements of the **Family File**

■ Access patients by name and chart number

■ Edit patient information such as, address and telephone number

Getting Started
Before you begin this assignment you may find it helpful to watch the Dentrix Learning Edition Videos' and the review the Dentrix User's Guide:

Dentrix Learning Edition Video

http://www.dentrix.com/le/on-demand-training

Family File

■ Viewing and Navigating the Family File

■ Quiz

User's Guide
Chapter 3: Family File

■ Windows Areas in Family File

■ The Tool Bar

■ Family Member List

Dentrix Practice

One of the key features of any practice management system is how patient files are managed. In the Dentrix Learning Edition program, this is done in the Family File. The Family File manages and stores both patient and family information, such as address, phone number, insurance coverage, and medical alerts. Before you can perfrom many of the functions you are required to select a patient.

Selecting a Patient

1. In the Family File, click the **Select Patient/New Family** button. The Select Patient dialogue box appears.

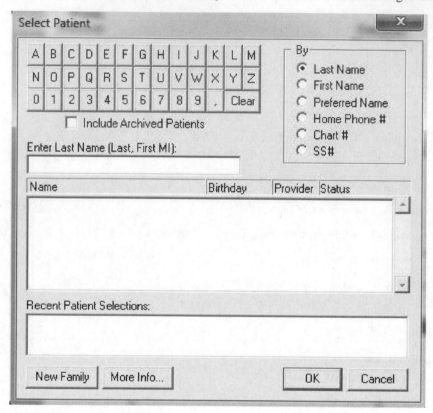

2. In the *by* group box, select the criteria for the search.

3. Enter the first few letters/numbers of the selected search method in the field provided.

4. Select the desired patient from the list.

5. Click **OK.**

Search for the following patients:

1. Alice Gleason

    a. What is Alice's chart number?

2. Chart #KE0004

    a. Who is the patient?

3. Henry Myers

    a. List the other family members.

Editing a Patient's File

1. In the Family File, click the **Select Patient/New Family** button. The Select Patient dialogue appears (see above).

2. In the *by* group box, select the criteria for the search.

3. Enter the first few letters/numbers of the selected search method in the field provided.

4. Select the desired patient from the list.

5. Click **OK.**

6. To edit information, double click in the block that contains the information you need to change.

   Edit the following information:

1. Karen Davis (head of household): New address (Double click on the address and bring up the Patient Information dialogue box.)
   36487 N. Shoreline Drive
   Eastside, NV 11111
   Note: Once a head of household address is changed, you will see a pop-up box that asks whether you want to change all family members.

2. Lisa Farrer: New address and phone
   7649 Lincoln Court
   Southside, NV 33333
   801-879-3210 (home)
   801-768-6554 (work)

3. Michael Smith: New address
   231897 Northwestern Avenue
   Centerville, NV 55555

DENTAL PRACTICE PROCEDURAL MANUAL PROJECT (OPTIONAL)

Continue working on your Dental Practice Procedural Manual (see Workbook Chapter 6 for details).
   Suggested activities:

- Team meeting

- Review timeline

- Review Group research and writing assignments

- Complete research and writing assignments for this chapter

- Review and revise completed sections of the manual

- Individual journal entries

8 Patient Clinical Records

LEARNING OBJECTIVES

1. List the functions of patient clinical records and the key elements of record keeping. Describe the significance of each element.
2. Explain the evolution of electronic clinical records in the dental office.
3. Identify the components of a clinical record and describe the function of each component.
4. Discuss methods used in the collection of information needed to complete clinical records.
5. Discuss the function of risk management and identify situations that lead to patient dissatisfaction.

INTRODUCTION

The function of the clinical record (paper or electronic) is to provide the dental healthcare team with information. The objective of the dental healthcare team is to deliver dental treatment that takes into consideration the needs of the patient. The whole picture cannot be correctly visualized if all of the pieces are not present. The information collected during preparation of the clinical record, when complete, provides all of the necessary pieces.

EXERCISES

1. List the functions of clinical records.

   _____

   _____

   _____

   _____

   _____

   _____

2. List the three manners in which electronic clinical records are created and stored.

   _____

   _____

   _____

3. List and describe the three HIPAA Security Standards that apply to electronic clinical records.

   _____

   _____

   _____

4. List the key elements of record keeping and describe the significance of each element.

_____

_____

_____

5. Provide two definitions of the term *accessibility* as it relates to clinical records.

_____

_____

6. Identify the components of a clinical record.

a. _____ Components of the clinical record are organized and placed inside.

b. _____ Provides demographic and financial information.

c. _____ Documents probing, bleeding, mobility, and furcation conditions.

d. _____ Outlines the work that is going to be done, describes reasonable results, and alerts the patient to complications that may result.

e. _____ Estimated cost of dental treatment and payment schedule.

f. _____ Necessary to document the medical needs as well as the dental needs of the patient.

g. _____ Used to update and record conditions at the time of each recall visit.

h. _____ Records treatment.

i. _____ Prioritizes treatment that needs to be performed.

j. _____ Logs letters sent and received.

k. _____ Authorizes release of information about the patient.

l. _____ Illustrates the current dental condition of the patient at the time he or she is first seen in the dental practice.

m. _____ Information about the patient's previous dental treatment.

n. _____ Plan derived from information collected in the clinical record.

A. Individual Patient File Folder

B. Treatment Plan Form

C. Telephone Information Form

D. Signature on File Form

E. Registration Form

F. Recall Examination Form

G. Progress Notes Form

H. Problem/Priority List

I. Periodontal Screening Examination Form

J. Medical History Form

K. Financial Arrangements Form

L. Dental Radiographs

M. Dental History Form

N. Correspondence Log

O. Consent Forms

P. Clinical Examination Form

Q. Acknowledgment of Receipt of Privacy Practices Notice

7. Identify the components of the patient clinical record that are necessary forms.

_____

_____

_____

_____

_____

8. Risk management is a process that

   a. organizes clinical records

   b. is mandated by state regulations

   c. identifies conditions that may lead to alleged malpractice

   d. is unnecessary in an organized dental practice

9. Major reason legal actions are decided in favor of the patient:

   a. A patient is right

   b. The dentist is guilty

   c. Dental assistant is unavailable to provide interpretation of clinical entries

   d. Poor record keeping

10. Characteristics of clinical record entries include all of the following except

    a. signature, date, and identification number of person making the entry

    b. use of standard abbreviations

    c. consistent line spacing

    d. marking an error and writing over

11. Which is an example of an objective statement?

    a. Mrs. Oliver is in a strange mood today; she wants to be seen only by Dr. Edwards.

    b. Mrs. Oliver said, "I want to see only Dr. Edwards today."

Preparing Clinical Records

Your assignment is to prepare a clinical record for four patients (information to follow). In each of the following chapters, you will be given an exercise that pertains to your patient and his or her clinical chart.

Step One: Select a method by which to organize your patient's clinical record. The objective is to maintain a separate record for each patient. You will need one of the following:

- Four lateral file folders, four fasteners (you can also staple the records)

- Four horizontal file folders, four fasteners

- One three-ring notebook, four dividers

Note: It is very important that you complete only the exercise assigned in each chapter.

Step Two: Prepare clinical records for the following patients using the blank forms supplied in the appendix at the back of this workbook (p. 108). Use the information given to complete the selected forms. Not all of the forms required for a clinical record will be included in the exercises. Where information is missing, leave the space blank.

12. Prepare a clinical record for Jana Rogers.

    Complete the following forms:

    - Registration Form

    - Clinical Examination Form

    - Treatment Plan Form

13. Prepare a clinical record for Angelica Green. Complete the following forms:

    - Registration Form

    - Medical and Dental Form

    - Clinical Examination Form

    - Periodontal Screening Form

    - Treatment Plan

14. Prepare a clinical record for Holly Barry. Select the forms you will need.

15. Prepare a clinical record for Lynn Bacca. Select the forms you will need.

JANA J. ROGERS
Patient Information

Patient .... Jana J. Rogers
Date of birth 3-12-2002
If child, parent name .... Donald Rogers
How do you wish to be addressed ....
Marital status .... Single
Home address .... 8176 Hillside
City .... Centerville
State/zip .... NV 55555
Business address ....
City ....
State/zip ....
Home phone 261-555-6217
Business phone ....
Patient/parent employer .... Valley Construction
Position .... Foreman
How long .... 12 yrs
Spouse/parent name .... Doris
Spouse employer .... Solutions Group
Position .... N/A
How long ....
Who is responsible for this account .... Donald Rogers
Driver's license number C3261
Method of payment .... Insurance
Purpose of call .... Toothache
Other members in this practice .... Donald, Doris, and Jason
Whom may we thank for this referral .... Parents
Notify in case of emergency .... Sadie Rogers
261-555-3001

Insurance Information 1st Coverage (Head of House)

Employee name .... Donald Rogers
Employee date of birth 2/8/64
Employer .... Valley Construction
Name of insurance co. .... Prudential
Address .... P.O. Box 15078
Albany, NY 12212-4094
Telephone 800-282-0555
Program or policy # 88442
Union local or group VC
Social Security # 012-34-5678
Fee Schedule .... None

Insurance Information 2nd coverage

Employee name .... Doris Rogers
Employee date of birth 12/2/67
Employer .... Solutions Group
Name of insurance co. .... Principal Financial Group
Address .... 10210 N 25th Ave, Phoenix, AZ 85021-3910
Telephone 800-328-8722
Program or policy # 88446
Union local or group .... Solutions Group
Social Security # 632-24-7654

50

Fee Schedule .... None
Provider .... Dennis Smith Jr.
Privacy request .... None
First visit 4/12/15

JANA J. ROGERS
Medical and Dental History Information

Medical information .... Normal (not necessary to complete for this exercise)
Allergies .... Penicillin
.... (enter in Med. Alert box on all appropriate forms for this patient)
Dental Information .... Normal (not necessary to complete for this exercise)

JANA J. ROGERS
Clinical Examination Information
Missing Teeth & Existing Restorations

2 .... MOD amalgam
13 .... O amalgam
14 .... B amalgam
18 .... DO amalgam
19 .... Sealant
30 .... MOD amalgam
1-16-17-32 .... Extracted
                                                                        Soft tissue examination okay
                                                                        Oral hygiene fair
                                                                        Calculus moderate
                                                                        Gingival bleeding none
                                                                        Perio exam no

Conditions/Treatment Indicated

3 .... DO amalgam
15 .... OB amalgam
18 .... B composite
30 .... Apical abscess/root canal
30 .... Core build-up (pre-fab)
30 .... PFM (high noble) crown

JANA J. ROGERS
Treatment Plan

Date	Category	Tooth #	Procedure	Fee
4/12	Diagnostic		Examination	35.00
	Preventive		Prophy a+110	60.00
	Diagnostic		4 bite-wing x-rays	40.00
	Diagnostic		1 PAs	16.00
5/17	Restorative	3	DO amalgam	85.00
5/17	Restorative	15	OB amalgam	85.00
4/24	Endodontic	30	Root canal	420.00
5/10	Endodontic	30	Post and core (pre-fab)	210.00
5/10	Restorative	30	PFM (high noble)	720.00
			Total Estimate	1671.00

All fees used in this exercise are for illustration only and do not represent actual fees charged for the procedures.

ANGELICA GREEN
Patient Information

Patient .... Angelica Green
Date of birth 7/20/87
If child, parent name ....
How do you wish to be addressed .... Angie
Marital status .... Married
Home address .... 724 E. Mark Ave
City .... Northside
State/zip .... NV 22222
Business address .... 3461 N. Cramer Ave
City .... Northside
State/zip .... NV 22222
Home phone 801-555-3004
Business phone 801-555-6134
Patient/parent employer .... James Taylor, DDS
Position .... RDA
How long .... 4 yrs
Spouse/parent name .... Anthony Green
Spouse employer .... Pacific States
Position .... Accountant
How long .... 8 yrs
Who is responsible for this account .... Anthony
Driver's license number 60314
Method of payment .... Insurance
Purpose of call .... Toothache
Other members in this practice .... None
Whom may we thank for this referral .... Dr. Taylor
Patient/parent SS # 736-82-9176
Spouse/parent SS # 286-34-2212
Notify in case of emergency .... Grace Miller, 801-555-9909

Insurance Information 1st Coverage (Head of House)

Employee name .... Anthony Green
Employee date of birth 9-13-87
Employer .... Pacific States
Name of Insurance co. .... Dental Select
Address .... 5373 S Green St
.... Salt Lake City UT 84123-5432
Telephone 800-999-9789
Program or policy # 95740
Union local or group .... Pacific States
Social Security # 286-34-2212
Fee Schedule   None

Employee name ....

Employee date of birth ....

Employer ....

Name of insurance co. ....

Address ....

Telephone ....

Program or policy # ....

Union local or group ....

Social Security # ....

Provider .... Paula Pearson

Privacy request .... No phone calls

First visit 3/6/15

ANGELICA GREEN
Medical and Dental History Information

Medical information .... Normal with following exceptions

Allergies .... Sulfa drugs and codeine (enter in Med. Alert box on all
appropriate forms for this patient)
Sensitive to latex
Bleeds easily when cut

Dental information .... Complete as much information as you can about the
patient

Aware of problem .... Bleeding gums when I brush

Clench and grind teeth .... Yes

Gums bleed .... Yes

ANGELICA GREEN
Clinical Examination Information
Missing Teeth & Existing Restoration

1 .... Missing

2 .... O composite

3 .... B composite

14 .... DO composite

16 .... Missing

17 .... Missing

32 .... Missing

Chief Complaint: Bleeding Gums

Soft tissue examination .... Normal

Oral hygiene .... Good

Calculus .... Heavy

Gingival bleeding .... General

Perio exam .... Yes

Conditions/Treatment Indicated

L/L .... Periodontal scaling and root planing

U/L .... Periodontal scaling and root planing

L/R .... Periodontal scaling and root planing

U/R .... Periodontal scaling and root planing

Periodontal Screening Examination

Tooth	Buccal	Lingual	Mobility	Furcation	Recession
2	676	455	1	2	1
3	876	767	1	2	1
4	444	444	0	0	0
14	876	765	1	2	1
15	453	543	1	2	1
18	547	665	1	1	0
19	767	878	1	1	0
30	455	445	1	1	0
31	667	778	1	1	0

ANGELICA GREEN
Treatment Plan

Date	Category	Tooth #	Procedure	Fee
3/6	Diagnostic		FMX	90.00
3/6	Diagnostic		Comprehensive exam	45.00
4/12	Perio	L/L	Periodontal scaling & root planing	175.00
4/12	Perio	U/L	Periodontal scaling & root planing	175.00
4/24	Perio	L/R	Periodontal scaling & root planing	175.00
4/24	Perio	U/R	Periodontal scaling & root planing	175.00
			Total Estimate	835.00

All fees used in this exercise are for illustration only and do not represent actual fees charged for the procedures.

HOLLY BARRY
Patient Information

Patient	Holly Barry
Date of birth	3/6/37
If child, parent name	NA
How do you wish to be addressed	Mrs. Barry
Marital status	Widowed
Home address	3264 S. Vine St
City	Westside
State/zip	NV 44444
Business address	NA
City	
State/zip	
Home phone	801-555-2331
Business phone	NA
Patient/parent employer	NA
Position	NA
How long	NA
Spouse/parent name	NA
Spouse employer	NA

Position .... NA
How long .... NA
Who is responsible for this account .... Self
Driver's license number 36788
Method of payment .... Credit Card
Purpose of call .... New Denture
Other members in this practice .... Son
.... Donald Rogers
Whom may we thank for this referral .... Donald
Patient/parent SS # 111-32-4356
Spouse/parent SS # .... NA
Notify in case of emergency .... Donald Rogers

Insurance Information 1st Coverage

Employee name .... NA
Employee date of birth .... NA
Employer .... NA
Name of insurance co. .... NA
Address .... NA
Telephone .... NA
Program or policy # .... NA
Union local or group .... NA
Social Security # .... NA

Insurance Information 2nd Coverage

Employee name .... NA
Employee date of birth .... NA
Employer .... NA
Name of insurance co. .... NA
Address .... NA
Telephone .... NA
Program or policy # .... NA
Union local or group .... NA
Social Security # .... NA
Provider .... Dennis Smith
Privacy request .... none
First visit 2/4
Fee Schedule   None

HOLLY BARRY
Medical and Dental History Information

Medical information .... Normal (not necessary to complete for this exercise)
Allergies .... NONE (enter in Med. Alert box on all appropriate forms for this patient)
SPECIAL NOTE .... Patient cannot sit for long periods of time, must get out of the dental chair and stretch every 60 minutes
Dental information .... Normal (not necessary to complete for this exercise)

HOLLY BARRY
Clinical Examination Information
Missing Teeth & Existing Restorations

1-16	Missing
17-19	Missing
29	MODLB Amalgam
U	Complete denture: Placed 1990, relined 3 times, loose fitting
L	Partial denture: Placed 1985, broken clasp

Chief complaint: Lower right molar broken
Upper denture very loose

Soft Tissue Examination	Normal
Oral Hygiene	Good
Calculus	Moderate
Gingival Bleeding	None
Perio Exam	Yes

Conditions/Treatment Indicated

U	Complete denture
29	PFM High noble
L	Partial denture, metal clasp, and framework

HOLLY BARRY
Treatment Plan

Date	Category	Tooth #	Procedure	Fee
2/4	Diagnostic		FMX	90.00
2/4	Diagnostic		Examination (limited)	35.00
4/12	Restorative	29	PFM	650.00
	Prostho		Complete maxillary denture	950.00
4/30	Prostho		Mandibular partial denture	
			Cast metal framework	1,050.00
			Total Estimate	2775.00

All fees used in this exercise are for illustration only and do not represent actual fees charged for the procedures.

LYNN BACCA
Patient Information

Patient	Lynn Bacca
Date of birth	8/12/2007
If child, parent name	Chuck Bacca
How do you wish to be addressed	Lynn
Marital status	Child
Home address	1812 Harman Dr
City	Southside
State/zip	NV 33333
Business address	34655 VIP Parkway
City	Westside
State/zip	NV 44444
Home phone	801-555-3421
Business phone	801-555-6210

Patient/parent employer	Diamond Welding
Position	Production Manager
How long	8 yrs
Spouse/parent name	Fern Bacca
Spouse employer	Columbia Healthcare
Position	Speech Pathologist
How long	5 yrs
Who is responsible for this account	Father
Driver's license number	878765
Method of payment	Insurance
Purpose of call	Exam
Other members in this practice	Parents, brother Steve
Whom may we thank for this referral	Aunt, Evelyn Evatt
	3245 S. Spring St
	Canyon View, CA 91711
Notify in case of emergency	Parent

Insurance Information 1st Coverage

Employee name	Chuck Bacca
Employee date of birth	7/27/82
Employer	Diamond Welding
Name of insurance co.	Delta Dental Plan
Address	PO Box 7736
	San Francisco CA 94120
Telephone	415-972-8300
Program or policy #	12121
Union local or group	Diamond
Social Security #	026-81-9217
Fee Schedule	None

Insurance Information 2nd Coverage

Employee name	Fern Bacca
Employee date of birth	7/5/85
Employer	Columbia Healthcare
Name of insurance co.	Connecticut General
Address	PO Box 1650
	Visalia, CA 93279
Telephone	800-252-2091
Program or policy #	55001
Union local or group	Columbia
Social Security #	213-90-7148
Fee Schedule	None
Provider	Brenda Childs
Privacy request	None
First visit	4/12

LYNN BACCA
Medical and Dental History Information

Medical information .... Normal (not necessary to complete for this exercise)

Allergies .... (enter in Med. Alert box on all appropriate forms for this patient)

Dental information .... Normal (not necessary to complete for this exercise)

LYNN BACCA
Clinical Examination Information
Missing Teeth and Existing Restorations

No Existing Restorations or Missing Teeth

Soft tissue examination .... Normal

Oral hygiene .... Good

Calculus .... None

Gingival bleeding .... None

Perio exam .... No

Conditions/Treatment Indicated

3 .... Sealant

14 .... Sealant

19 .... Sealant

30 .... Sealant

LYNN BACCA
Treatment Plan

Date	Category	Tooth #	Procedure	Fee
4/12	Diagnostic		BW x-Rays (4)	40.00
	Diagnostic		2 ANT PA's	14.00
	Preventive		Prophy and Fluoride TX	54.00
4/24	Preventive	3	Sealant	32.00
	Preventive	14	Sealant	32.00
	Preventive	19	Sealant	32.00
	Preventive	30	Sealant	32.00
			Total Estimate	236.00

All fees used in this exercise are for illustration only and do not represent actual fees charged for the procedures.

DENTRIX EXERCISES

Dentrix Learning Objective

- Create a Family File for new patients and their families.

- Enter important patient information, such as patient demographics, medical alerts, and employer and insurance information.

- Create and print a pre-treatment plan.

Getting Started

Before you begin this assignment you may find it helpful to watch the Dentrix Learning Edition Videos' and review the Dentrix User's Guide:

Dentrix Learning Edition Video

http://www.dentrix.com/le/on-demand-training

Family File

- Adding Patient and Family Information

- Quiz

Insurance Management

- Adding Patient and Family Information

- Quiz

Ledger

- Viewing and Navigating the Ledger

User's Guide

Chapter 3: Family File

    Adding a New Family (Account)

    Adding Family Members

    Assigning Medical Alerts

    Assigning Employers

    Insurance Information

Insurance Information

Multiple Coverage Dental Insurance Plans

Chapter 8: Ledger

    Ledger Overview

    Working with Treatment Plans

Creating a family file

To add a new family into the Learning Edition, you must create a file for the head-of-house. Once the head-of-house has been entered, you can add each additional family member to the family. *Note:* If the head-of-house is not a patient, change the status from *patient* to *nonpatient* (located in the drop down menu in the *Status* field). For detailed information on how to complete the Head-of-House Information box, refer to the Dentrix *User's Guide,* Family File—Adding a New Family (Account).

To create a file for the head-of-house:

1. In the Family File, click the **Select Patient/New Family** button. The Select Patient dialogue box appears.

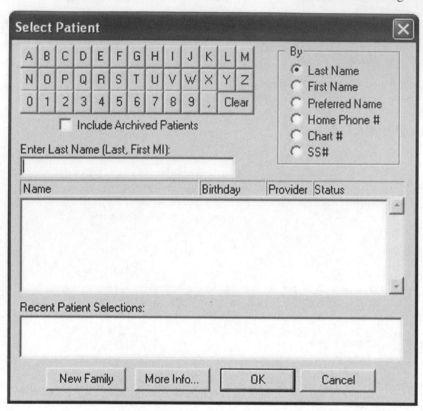

2. Click **New Family**. The Head-of House Information dialogue box appears.

Head-of-House Information

Name
Last   First   MI   Preferred

Salutation   Title   ☐ Print Title on Stmts

Status
Patient ▾   Male ▾   Single ▾

Personal
Birthdate   Age   SS#   Other ID

Driver's License #

Address
Street

City   ST   Zip

E-Mail

Phone
Home   Work   Ext.   Time To Call

FAX   Mobile   Other

Office
Prov1   Prov2
>>   >>

Fee Schedule
<NONE>   >>

Chart
<AUTO>   >>

Consent
04/20/2015

Privacy Requests
☐ No phone calls
☐ No correspondence
☐ Disclosure restrictions

Visits
First Visit   Last Visit
04/20/2015

Last Missed   #
Appt   Missed
0

OK   Cancel

(*Note:* The Head-of-House and the Patient Information dialogue boxes have the same fields, but the titles are different to inform you to enter the head-of-house's or new family member's information.)

2. Click **New Family**. The Head-of-House Information dialog box appears

3. Enter the patient's or head-of house's name in the Name group box.

   For this exercise use the information for Angelica Green (page 45). *Hint:* Anthony Green is the Head of Household.

4. Enter the patient's or head-of house's name in the *Name* group box.

5. Enter a salutation (this will appear on letters you create), such as Dear Mr. Green

6. Enter a title (optional)

7. In the *Status group* box, select the patient status (for Mr. Green it is non-patient), gender, and marital status.

8. In the *Personal group* box, enter the birth date, Social Security number, and driver's license number.

9. In the *Other* field in the Personal group box is used on some insurance forms when a separate patient ID is required to file a claim.

10. In the *Address* group box, enter the street address, zip code, and email address in the corresponding fields.

11. In the *Office* group box, select the primary and secondary providers (DDS1)

12. Select the option in the *Privacy Request* group box if applicable.

13. Click **OK** to save and add the head-of-house to the database.

Adding Family Members

Follow these steps after you have entered all the information related to the head-of-house:

1. Click the **Add Family Member** button on the toolbar. The Patient Information dialogue box appears. The last name, provider, home phone number, and address default to the information entered for the head-of-house file.

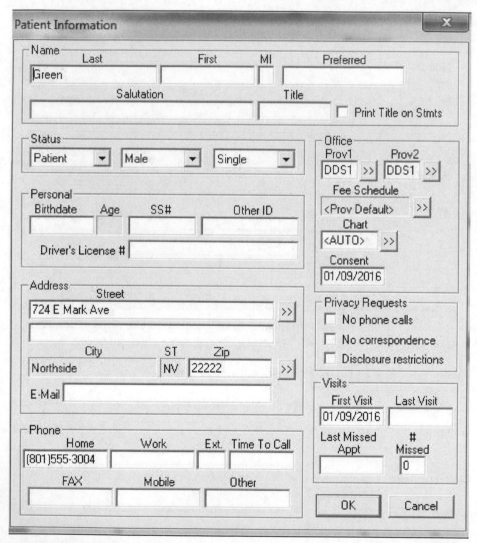

2. Enter Family member information (Angelica Green) in the appropriate field. Hint: Check Angelica's information carefully, she has a different provider and privacy request.

3. Click OK

Note: Refer to the Dentrix User's Guide Family File–Adding a new Family section for a complete explanation of each field.

Assigning Medical Alerts to Patient

Once you have created a file for a patient in the Family File, you may need to assign medical alerts to the patient. To assign medical alerts to a patient:

1. In the Family File, select a patient (Angelica Green)

2. Double click the **Medical Alerts** block. The Medical Alerts dialog appears.

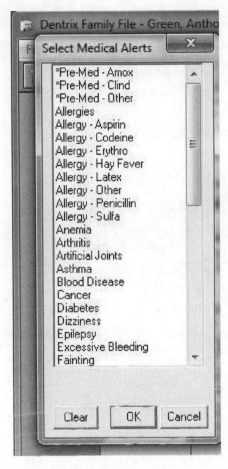

3. Click **Edit**. The Select Medical Alerts dialog appears.

4. Select all of the alert(s) to assign to the patient.

5. Click **OK** to return to the Medical Alerts dialog.

6. Click **Close** to return to the Family File.

Assigning an Employer to the Patient

1. In the Family File, select a patient (Angelica Green)

2. Double click the **Employer** Block. The Employer Information dialog appears

3. In the **Employer Name** field, enter the first few letters of the patient's employer.

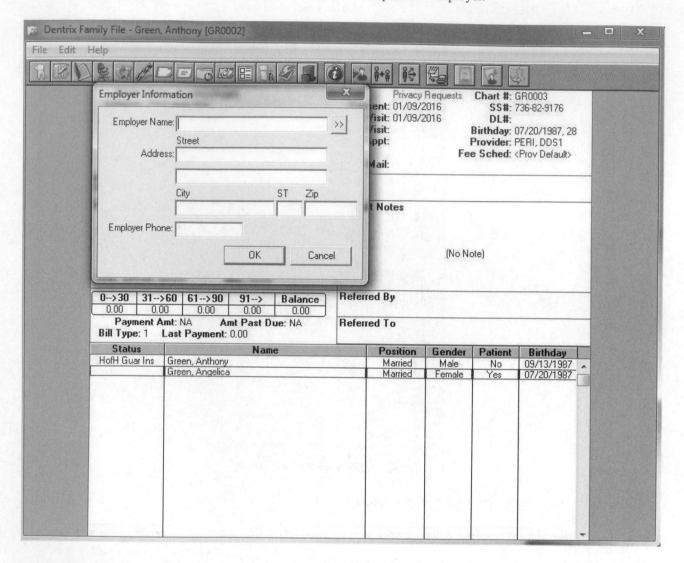

4. Click the **Employer Name** search button to determine whether the employer is already in the database to help avoid duplicates. The Select Employer dialog appears.

5. Select the employer or enter the employer's information. Note: If the employer's information is not listed click **Cancel** to return to the Employer Information dialog and complete the fields.

6. Click **OK** to return to the Family File

Chapter **8 Patient Clinical Records**

Assigning Insurance

Note: To assign insurance to a patient, the insurance subscriber must be listed as a family member in the patient's Family File. If the subscriber is not a patient, set the status to *Nonpatient* in the subscriber's patient information and complete the insurance information.

Assigning Primary Insurance to a Patient

1. From the Family File, select the patient/subscriber.

2. Double click the **Insurance Information** block. The Insurance Information dialogue box appears. Select the subscriber of the insurance (Anthony Green).

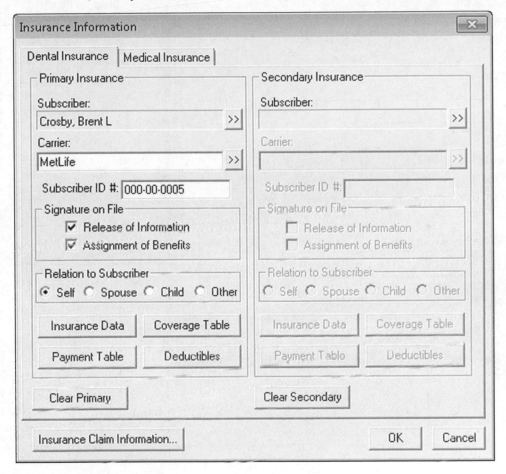

3. Click the **Carrier** search button. (≫) The Select Primary Dental Insurance Plan dialog appears.

4. In the *Search By* group box, mark the desired search method.

5. Enter the first few letters/numbers of the selected search method in the field provided.

6. Select the desired plan. If the plan is not listed, follow the steps outlined in the *Adding a New Insurance Plan* in the *User's Guide*. If the plan is listed, select the plan from the list and click **OK** to return to the Insurance Information dialog box.

7. Verify that the subscriber ID number is correct (add the information if missing).

8. Verify that the correct options are checked in the *Signature on File* group box.

9. Verify that the correct option is marked in the *Relation to Subscriber* group box.

10. Click **OK** to return to the Family File.

Assigning Primary Insurance to a Patient (non-subscriber)

1. From the Family File, select the patient (Angelica Green).

2. Double click the **Insurance Information** block. The Insurance Information dialogue box appears.

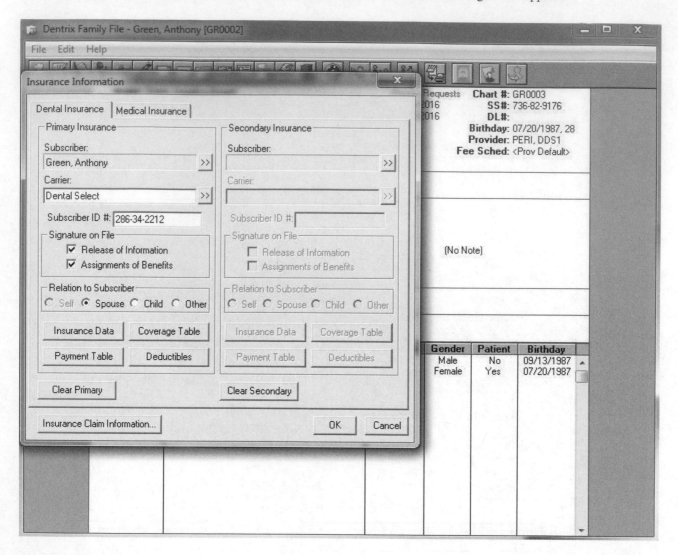

3. Click the **Search** button (≫) next to **Subscriber.** The Select Primary Subscriber dialogue box appears.

4. Select the primary subscriber and click **OK** to return to the Insurance Information dialogue box. *Note:* If the subscriber is not listed, you will need to add him or her as a patient and assign insurance information before you can continue.

5. Select **Release of Information** and **Assignments of Benefits.**

6. Select Self, Spouse, Child, or Other as the patient's relation to the subscriber.

7. If the patient has secondary insurance coverage, enter the information in the *Secondary Insurance* box.

8. Click **OK** to return to the Family File.

Creating a Pretreatment Estimate

1. Click the **Select Patient** button on the Ledger toolbar. Enter the first few letters of the patient's last name (Angelica Green). Select the desired patient and click **OK.** *Note:* If you have the patient's file open in Family File, select the Ledger button from the toolbar; this will open the patient's ledger.

2. From the Ledger menu bar, select Options, then Treatment Plan. *Note:* The Ledger Title Bar now reflects that you are in the Treatment Plan View.

3. To add procedures, click the **Enter Procedure** button on the Ledger toolbar. The Enter Procedure(s) dialogue box appears.

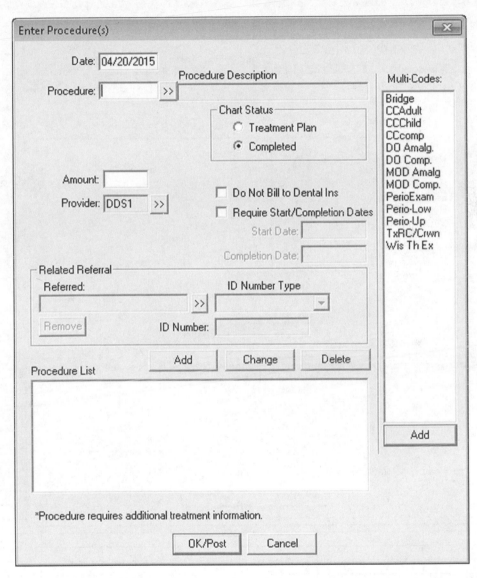

Add procedures to the Procedure list using individual codes or selecting the search button. Select the appropriate ADA Category. All procedure codes assigned to that category are displayed in the Procedure List. Select the desired code and click **OK.**

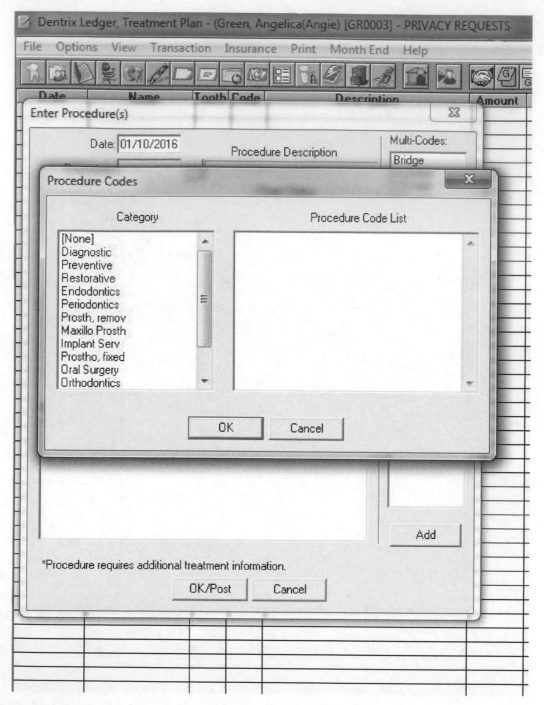

4. If the procedure code requires additional treatment information such as surface, tooth number, or quadrant, you should enter those now.

5. Once a procedure code has been selected a fee will be automatically assigned according to the fee schedule on file. However, you can enter a different fee in the **Amount** field.

6. Click **Add** to add this procedure to the Procedure Pane.

7. Repeat steps 1 through 6 for all procedures.

8. When all procedures have been listed click **OK/POST.**

9. To print the Treatment Plan click the **Treatment Planner** button on the Ledger toolbar. This will open the Treatment Planner window. For additional information on how to use the functions of the Treatment Planner refer to Chapter 5 in the User's Guide and view the on-demand-videos.

10. Click **File > Print > Treatment Case**

Dentrix Application

For this exercise, you will use the same information you used to create clinical records for Jana Rogers, Angelica Green, Holly Barry, and Lynn Bacca.

1. Prepare a Family File for the Rogers family.

   A. Create a New Family with Donald Rogers as head-of-house.

   Note: Assign subscriber insurance information by double clicking on the Insurance Information Block (see directions above).

   B. Add Doris as a new family member (see directions above to assign subscriber insurance information).

   C. Add Jana as a new family member (see directions above to assign insurance).

   D. Create a pretreatment estimate for Jana (see directions above).

2. Prepare a Family File for the Green family. You have completed the majority of this assignment during the Dentrix Practice exercise. Review the file and check for completeness.

   A. Create a New Family with Anthony Green as H/H. (*Note:* Anthony is not a patient.) Assign subscriber insurance information.

   B. Add Angelica as a new family member and assign insurance.

   C. Create a pretreatment estimate for Angelica.

3. Prepare a Family File for Holly Barry.

   A. Create a New Family with Holly as H/H and patient.

   B. Create a pretreatment estimate for Holly.

4. Prepare a Family File for the Bacca family.

   A. Create a New Family with Chuck as H/H. Assign subscriber insurance information.

   B. Add Fern as a new family member and assign subscriber insurance information.

   C. Add Lynn as a new family member.

5. Check the total estimate for each patient on the worksheet in the workbook. Do the figures match the total estimate on the patient's treatment plan? (*Hint:* If the totals do not match, did you change the fee when entering the procedure information?) Correct any figures that are not correct. Print out a copy of each patient's treatment plan. (Jana, Angelica and Holly) and place in the patients clinical record.

Dentrix Charting

If you completed the charting exercises in Chapter 2 and would like additional practice charting, use the Patient Chart module to enter the treatment for the above patients. Use the information provided in the Clinical Exam Information and Treatment Plan for each patient (information was provided earlier in this chapter of the workbook.)

DENTAL PRACTICE PROCEDURAL MANUAL PROJECT (OPTIONAL)

Continue working on your Dental Practice Procedural Manual (see Workbook Chapter 6 for details).
  Suggested activities:

- Team meeting

- Review timeline

- Review Group research and writing assignments

- Complete research and writing assignments for this chapter

- Review and revise completed sections of the manual

- Individual journal entries

9 | Information Management

LEARNING OBJECTIVES

1. List and describe the six filing methods outlined in this chapter, including demonstration of the ARMA (a not-for-profit professional organization and the authority on management of records and information) Simplified Filing Standard Rules.
2. Compare and contrast the filing methods used for business records such as accounts payable and personnel records versus patient and insurance information.
3. List and describe types of filing equipment to store information for a paper system.
4. List and describe filing supplies, including types of file labels.
5. Prepare a new patient's clinical record for filing.
6. Prepare a business document for filing (manually and electronically).
7. Discuss how long records must be retained and the two methods of transferring records.

INTRODUCTION

The responsibilities of the administrative dental assistant in the management of information and records are multifaceted. In today's dental practice, the storage of information may involve both paper files and electronic files. Although methods of documentation may vary, the principles of a records management program will always be the same. According to the International Organization for Standardization (ISO), in *Information and Documentation—Records Management,* a general policy should involve "... the creation and management of authentic, reliable and useable records, capable of supporting business function and activities for as long as they are required." The importance of collecting the correct information and preparation of a dental record was discussed in Chapter 8. This chapter discusses basic methods used in a systematic approach to the storage and retrieval of information (filing).

EXERCISES

1. What is the main purpose of managing documents and information in a dental practice?

2. List the six basic filing methods and give an example of how they may be used in a dental practice.

_____

_____

_____

_____

_____

3. Explain the order in which electronic records are organized.

4. Using the personal name rule, identify which information will be placed in the following:

Unit 1 _____

Unit 2 _____

Unit 3 _____

Unit 4 _____

5. Using the business rule, identify which information will be placed in the following:

Unit 1 _____

Unit 2 _____

Unit 3 _____

Unit 4 _____

6. When a numeric filing system is used for patient records, a key component in locating the record is

   a. charts are arranged numerically

   b. charts are color-coded

   c. charts are randomly assigned numbers

   d. charts are cross-referenced

7. Geographic category records are filed according to

   a. ZIP code

   b. area code

   c. city

   d. state

   e. all of the above

8. Subject filing is a method of filing strictly by subject. True or false, and why?

   _____

   _____

   _____

9. Which method indexes by date?

   _____

10. **Matching:** Identify the method of filing that would be used when a system is established for the following types of business documents. If a system uses two methods, list the primary location first, and the secondary method second. For example: Personnel files are first filed by subject (S) (primary location) and then filed alphabetically (A) by employee (secondary method). The answer will be S/A.

a. ___/___Accounts payable   S. Subject

b. ___/___Accounts receivable (ledger)   G. Geographic

c. ___/___Bank statements   A. Alphabetical

d. ___/___Financial reports   N. Numerical

e. ___/___Personnel records   C. Chronological

f. ___/___Payroll records

g. ___/___Tax records

h. ___/___Business reports

i. ___/___Insurance reports (business)

j. ___/___Insurance claims (patient)

k. ___/___Professional correspondence

l. ___/___Patient information

11. Maintaining an active filing system requires the removal of inactive records and documents. Identify two types of transfer methods and briefly describe how each method works.

_____

_____

_____

_____

12. List the six basic rules for properly indexing names for filing.

_____

_____

_____

_____

_____

_____

_____

_____

_____

ACTIVITY EXERCISE

Complete the preparation of clinical records by preparing a file label for the following patients. Follow the guidelines listed in the text. (See Anatomy of an Indexed File Folder, p. 144.)

13. Jana Rogers

14. Angelica Green

15. Holly Barry

16. Lynn Bacca

WHAT WOULD YOU DO?

You have been asked to write the new office policy for safeguarding patients' clinical records (paper or electronic, your choice). You will need to research HIPAA policy and procedures. How will this be applied to a dental office?

1. Identify the type of records you will be addressing in your procedure guide (electronic or paper).

2. Research the HIPAA Policy for your selected choice.

3. Write a HIPAA Procedures Guide to be used in a dental office.

DENTAL PRACTICE PROCEDURAL MANUAL PROJECT (OPTIONAL)

Continue working on your Dental Practice Procedural Manual (see Workbook Chapter 6 for details).
Suggested activities:

- Team meeting

- Review timeline

- Review Group research and writing assignments

- Complete research and writing assignments for this chapter

- Review and revise completed sections of the manual

- Individual journal entries

10 Dental Patient Scheduling

LEARNING OBJECTIVES

1. Describe the mechanics of scheduling, including the criteria required for matrixing an electronic scheduler or manual appointment book.
2. Discuss the art of scheduling and how to maximize scheduling efficiency, including the different methods used to identify when specific procedures should be scheduled.
3. Explain the seven different scenarios of appointment scheduling and formulate an action plan to solve the problems.
4. Describe the four ways that patients may schedule an appointment, including the use of traditional and alternative types of appointment cards and reminders.
5. Explain how use of a call list and daily schedule sheets can save time in the dental office.
6. List the steps to be followed in performing the daily routine associated with the appointment schedule.

INTRODUCTION

Developing and implementing an organized, functional schedule for a dental practice requires time, experience, and the cooperation of the entire dental healthcare team. The process of scheduling appointments involves more than entering names in a book or keying them into a computer. Scheduling is a complex process that has two main elements. The first is the mechanics of scheduling, which includes selecting the appointment book (manual or electronic), outlining or matrixing, and entering information.

EXERCISES

1. If an appointment book has four time slots per hour, each time slot represents _____.

    a. 10 minutes

    b. 15 minutes

    c. 20 minutes

    d. 30 minutes

2. The dentist tells you that Judy will need 9 units for her next appointment (you are scheduling at 10-minute intervals). How long will Judy's appointment be?

    a. 1 hour

    b. 1 hour 10 minutes

    c. 1 hour 20 minutes

    d. 1 hour 30 minutes

3. A column in an appointment book is assigned to

    a. an individual practitioner

    b. a treatment room

    c. be used for information

    d. all of the above

4. List the four steps involved in scheduling a follow-up appointment for a patient.

_____

_____

_____

_____

5. Place the following tasks in order. Place the number 1 in front of the first task to be completed, 2 before the second, and so on.

   a. _____ Check patients' charts for any information that may not have been included on the schedule, such as need for premedication, payments due, or updated insurance and medical information.

   b. _____ Confirm or remind patients of their upcoming appointments.

   c. _____ Confirm the return of laboratory work.

   d. _____ Give patients' clinical records to the dental assisting staff to review before they see the patients.

   e. _____ Keep the dental healthcare team and patients informed of any changes that will affect their schedules.

   f. _____ Pull the patients' clinical records, and review the procedures that are going to be completed the following day.

   g. _____ Spend 5 to 10 minutes with the dental healthcare team to review the daily schedule.

   h. _____ Type the daily schedule (or print out from the computer).

   i. _____ Update schedules throughout the day as changes occur.

   j. _____ Use the call list to fill any openings in the day's schedule.

6. List the criteria for making an appointment book entry. (See Anatomy of an Appointment Book, p. 153).

_____

_____

_____

_____

_____

_____

ACTIVITY EXERCISE

You will need the clinical records you have completed for the following patients:

Jana Rogers

Angelica Green

Holly Barry

Lynn Bacca

7. Matrix an appointment book page (see p. 64) for one day, April 12. There are four dentists and an expanded function dental assistant (EFDA) who have patients. How can you design the daily schedule so that each dentist does not have to share the treatment room with another provider while in the office? Use the following criteria:

   a. Three columns: treatment room one, treatment room two, and treatment room three

   b. 15-minute intervals

   c. Include a 15-minute buffer period for emergencies for each dentist.

8. Schedule your patients. Check your patients' clinical records for detailed information on work to be completed on April 12 (treatment plan).

Jana Rogers	4 units with Dr. Dennis Smith Jr.
Angelica Green	8 units with Dr. Paula Pearson
Holly Barry	3 units with Dr. Dennis Smith
	2 units with EFDA for temporary crown
Lynn Bacca	2 units with Dr. Brenda Childs
	3 units with EFDA for coronal polish and fluoride treatment

(Review Anatomy of an Appointment Book, p. 153 in textbook.)

9. Complete a Daily Schedule for April 12.

	Treatment Room 1	Treatment Room 2	Treatment Room 3
8 00			
15			
30			
45			
9 00			
15			
30			
45			
10 00			
15			
30			
45			
11 00			
15			
30			
45			
12 00			
15			
30			
45			
1 00			
15			
30			
45			
2 00			
15			
30			
45			
3 00			
15			
30			
45			
4 00			
15			
30			
45			
5 00			
15			
30			
45			
6 00			
15			
30			
45			

10. Complete an appointment card for each patient.

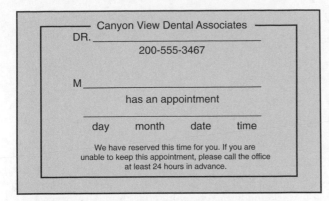

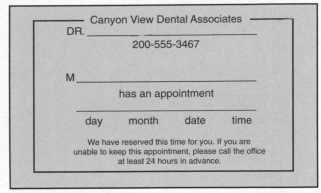

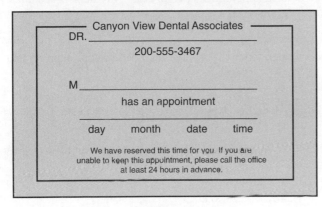

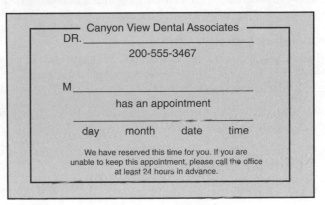

Dentrix Learning Objectives

■ Set up the practice schedule.

■ Determine available appointment times.

■ Schedule appointments for patients.

Getting Started

Before you begin this assignment you may find it helpful to watch the Dentrix Learning Edition Videos' and review the Dentrix User's Guide:

Dentrix Learning Edition Video

http://www.dentrix.com/le/on-demand-training

Appointment Book

    Viewing and Navigating the Appointment Book

    Quiz

    Setting Up Your Schedule

    Quiz

    Scheduling and Completing Appointments

Dentrix User's Guide

Using Appointment Book

Setting Up Appointment Book

View Options Overview

Scheduling Appointments (quick start and scheduling treatment plan views)

Changing Schedule Hours

Appointment Book Tips and Tricks

DENTRIX PRACTICE

The Dentrix Appointment Book (or any electronic scheduler) is an essential component of the practice management software program. The electronic appointment book allows you to track appointments; color code providers, procedures, and operatories; print route slips; and communicate vital patient information.

Operatory Setup

Before you begin it will be necessary to determine the number of operatories that will be included in your appointment book. For this exercise you will be using 5 operatories.

To delete unused operatories:

1. In the Office Manager, select **Maintenance—Practice Setup—Practice Resource Setup**. The Practice Resource Setup dialog box appears.

2. In the Operatories group box, select the operatory you would like to delete and click **Delete.** Repeat until you have a total of 5 operatories.

3. Click **Close.**

Setting Up the Appointment Book

The **Practice Appointment Setup** options in Appointment Book allow you to customize your practice hours, some appointment defaults, and the time block size used.

To set up practice hours:

1. In Appointment Book, from the **Setup** menu, click **Practice Appointment Setup.** The **Practice Appointment Setup** dialogue box appears.

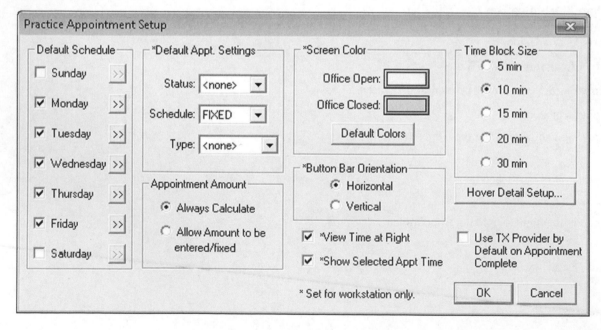

2. Dentrix allows you to schedule your appointments in 5-minute, 10-minute, 15-minute, 20-minute, or 30-minue intervals. Click the **Time Block Size.** (*Note:* In this exercise it will be a 15-minute interval.)

3. Dentrix defaults to a Monday through Friday workweek.

    a. Select the days of the week the office is usually open. (*Note:* For this exercise the office is open Monday through Friday.)

    b. Clear the days the office is closed.

4. You can set working hours for each selected day.

    a. Click the **search** button (≫) to the right of the day.

    b. To change the time range for a time block, click the Start Time or End Time **Search** button (≫) of the time block you want to change.

    Note: For this exercise, set the following times:

Monday	8:00 AM to 12:00 PM and 1:00 PM to 5:00 PM
Tuesday	8:00 AM to 12:00 PM and 1:30 PM to 5:30 PM
Wednesday	10:00 AM to 2:00 PM and 2:30 pm to 8:00 PM
Thursday	10:00 AM to 2:00 PM and 2:30 PM to 8:00 PM
Friday	10:00 AM to 1:00 PM and 1:15 PM to 3:00 PM

    c. When finished click **OK.**

5. Specify the default settings you want the Appointment Book to use for each new appointment when it is created.

    a. Set the default **Status** field to **??????.**

    b. Set the default **Schedule** field to **Fixed.**

    c. Set the default **Type** field to **General.**

6. Under **Appointment Amount** for this exercise, select **Always Calculate.**

7. (Optional). Set the colors you want Appointment Book to display.

8. Select **Button Bar Orientation, Horizontal** or **Vertical.**

9. Select **View Time at Right.**

10. Click **OK.**

Setting Up Providers
To set up the provider hours:

1. In Appointment Book, from the **Setup** menu, click **Provider Setup.**

2. Select the provider for whom you want to set a schedule. For this exercise select DDS1 (Dr. Dennis Smith).

3. Click **Setup.**

The **Provider Setup** dialogue box appears.

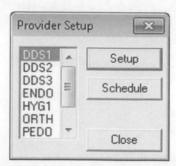

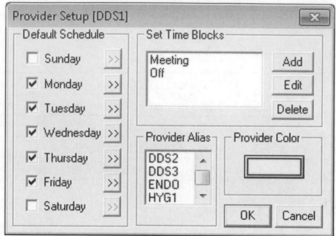

4. Select the days of the week the provider usually works.

5. Set the working hours for each selected day.

   You can set working hours for each selected day.

   a. Click the **search** button (≫) to the right of the day.

   b. To change the time range for a time block, click the Start Time or End Time **Search** button (≫) of the time block you want to change.

   Note: For this exercise, set the following times:

Monday	8:00 am-12:00 pm and 1:00 pm-5:00 pm
Tuesday	8:00 am-12:00 pm and 1:30 pm to 5:30 pm
Wednesday	10:00 am-2:00 pm and 2:30 pm to 8:00 pm
Thursday	10:00 am-2:00 pm and 2:30 pm to 8:00 pm
Friday	10:00 am-1:00 pm and 1:15 pm to 3:00 pm

   c. When finished click **OK**.

6. If desired, edit the provider's appointment book color in the Provider Color group box by clicking the color button.

7. Click **OK** to save changes.

8. Click **Close** to return to the Appointment Book.

   Repeat this process to setup the following providers:

   DDS2 (Dr. Dennis Smith, Jr.)

PEDO (Dr. Brenda Childs)

HYG1 (Sally Hayes)

Scheduling Appointments

Scheduling appointments can be done in several different ways depending on the type and complexity of the appointment (for a full description refer to the Dentrix User's Guide).

Scheduling (quick start)

The following instructions explain the simplest way to schedule an appointment.

1. Either by manually finding an appointment time or by using the Dentrix Find feature (discussed in the Dentrix *User's Guide*), locate and open schedule space.

2. In the Appointment Book, double click the appropriate operatory at the time you want to schedule the appointment. The **Select Patient** dialogue box appears.

3. Enter the first few letters of the patient's last name (Green).

4. Select the patient you want from the list (Angelica Green), and then click **OK.** The **Appointment Information** dialogue box appears. The **Provider** field defaults to the patient's primary provider.

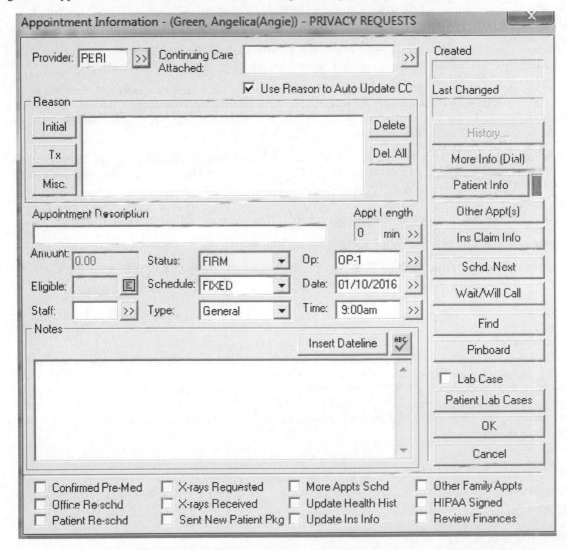

5. If necessary, click the **Provider** search button (≫) to select another provider for the appointment. (Select HYG1 as the provider.)

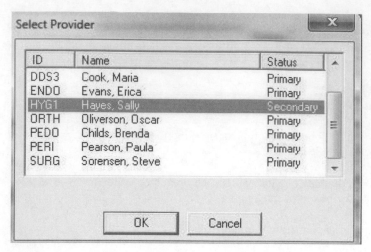

6. Under **Reason,** select a reason for the appointment using any of the following methods:

   a. If you are seeing the patient for work that would be done on an initial visit, such as an exam or a cleaning, click **Initial.** In the **Select Initial Reasons** dialogue box, select the reasons for the appointment and then click **OK.**

   b. If you are seeing the patient for a treatment that was previously planned, click **Tx.** In the **Treatment Plan** dialogue box, select the reasons for the appointment (Periodontal Scaling), and then click **Close.**

   c. To add a new treatment-planned procedure, click **New Tx.** In the **Enter Procedure(s)** dialogue box, click the **Procedure** search button (≫), select the procedures you want from the **Procedure Codes** dialogue box, and then click **OK.** In the **Enter Procedure(s)** dialogue box, click **OK/Post.** In the **Treatment Plan** dialogue box, select the procedure you want for the appointment and click **Close.**

   d. If you are seeing the patient for a treatment that has not been planned, click **Misc.** In the **Procedure Codes** dialogue box, select a **Category** from the list; under **Procedure Code List,** select the procedure code you want, and then click **OK.**

7. Once you have entered a reason, Dentrix automatically assigns a length of time to the appointment.

   a. To change the length, click the **Appt Length** search button ≫.

   b. In the **Appointment Time Pattern** dialogue box, click the right arrow to increase or the left arrow to decrease the number of minutes needed, and then click **OK.**

8. Click **OK** to save any changes you have made and close the **Appointment Information** dialogue box.

Dentrix Application

For this exercise you will schedule the appointments listed below. Schedule all the patients for the same day. *Note:* You have already set up treatment plans for Jana Rogers, Angelica Green, and Holly Barry. Determine the provider from the list of providers that you have setup (DDS1, DDS2, HYG1 or PEDO). Decide ahead of time whether you will be assigning an operatory to specific providers. For example, does the hygienist work out of one predetermined operatory? Are there specific operatories assigned to the different providers? Refer to Scheduling (quick start) above for directions on scheduling your patients.

1. Jana Rogers (1 hour)

   a. Examination

   b. Prophy

   c. 4-bite wing x-rays

2. Angelica Green (2 hours)

   a. Periodontal Scaling (L/L & U/L)

3. Mrs. Barry (2.5 hours)

   a. PFM (tooth #29)

   b. Final Impressions for maxillary denture

4. Lynn Bacca (*Note:* You will need to check Lynn's paper chart for fees.)

   a. 4-bite wing x-rays

   b. 2 anterior PAs

   c. Prophy and Fluoride Treatment

DENTAL PRACTICE PROCEDURAL MANUAL PROJECT (OPTIONAL)

Continue working on your Dental Practice Procedural Manual (see Workbook Chapter 6 for details).
Suggested activities:

- Team meeting
- Review timeline
- Review Group research and writing assignments
- Complete research and writing assignments for this chapter
- Review and revise completed sections of the manual
- Individual journal entries

11 Recall Systems

11

LEARNING OBJECTIVES

1. Define recall system, and explain the benefits of a continuing care (recall) program for patients and the financial health of a dental practice, including the elements that are necessary for an effective recall system.
2. List the different classifications of recalls.
3. Identify the methods for recalling patients and explain the barriers and solutions for each method.

INTRODUCTION

A **recall system** is an organized method of scheduling patients for examinations, prophylaxis, or other dental treatments. The success of a recall system is dependent on several factors: (1) Patients must be willing to return to the dental practice for follow-up care and examinations. (2) The dental practice must follow the procedure consistently to schedule patients at the prescribed time. (3) The dental practice must have an efficient method for tracking and contacting patients who fail to return at the scheduled time.

EXERCISES

1. The success of a recall system is dependent on three factors. Identify these factors.

_____

_____

_____

2. List the benefits to the patient of a recall appointment.

_____

_____

_____

_____

_____

_____

_____

3. List the benefits to the dental practice of a recall system.

_____

_____

_____

_____

_____

_____

4. During a recall appointment, the dentist has the opportunity to reexamine the patient and evaluate his or her dental health. Identify other treatments besides prophylaxis that may require a recall appointment.

_____

_____

_____

_____

_____

_____

5. Identify the following methods of recalling patients:

a. _____ This method is highly successful because patients have personally participated in the scheduling of their own appointment.

b. _____ Requires the mailing of recall cards to patients to remind them that they are due in the dental office for an appointment.

c. _____ Requires an assistant to call each patient before the month they are due for recall to schedule the appointment.

d. _____ Forms a partnership with the patient, and the recall appointment is worked around his or her preference.

A. Combination Recall System

B. Mail Recall System

C. Prescheduled Recall System

D. Telephone Recall System

E. Tracking System

WHAT WOULD YOU DO?

During a recent staff meeting, several issues have been raised about the effectiveness of the current recall system. The dental healthcare team has identified the following concerns:

- The hygiene schedule is booked 3 months in advance.

- There has been a decline in new patients.

- Patients are not responding to the reminder postcards that are being sent.

6. Your task as the administrative assistant is to evaluate these concerns by identifying the problem and presenting a possible solution. You will present your findings in the form of a report at your next staff meeting.

_____

_____

_____

_____

_____

_____

_____

_____

_____

_____

_____

_____

_____

DENTRIX EXERCISE (OPTIONAL)

Dentrix Learning Objectives
■ Assign a continuing care plan

Getting Started
Before you begin this assignment you may find it helpful to watch the Dentrix Learning Edition Videos' and review the Dentrix User's Guide:

Dentrix Learning Edition Video

http://www.dentrix.com/le/on-demand-training

Dentrix User's Guide
Assigning Continuing Care (Recall)

Editing and Existing Continuing Care Type

Clearing an Existing Continuing Care Type

Dentrix allows the use of multiple Continuing Care types (recall information). Review the information in the Dentrix *User's Guide*, Family File, section titled "Assigning Continuing Care."

7. Assign a continuing care plan for Jana Rogers, Angelica Green, Holly Barry, and Lynn Bacca.

DENTAL PRACTICE PROCEDURAL MANUAL PROJECT (OPTIONAL)

Continue working on your Dental Practice Procedural Manual (see Workbook Chapter 6 for details).
Suggested activities:

- Team meeting

- Review timeline

- Review Group research and writing assignments

- Complete research and writing assignments for this chapter

- Review and revise completed sections of the manual

- Individual journal entries

12 Inventory Management

LEARNING OBJECTIVES

1. Explain how to establish a successful inventory management system, including:
   - List the information needed to order supplies and products and discuss how this information will be used.
   - Define *rate of use* and *lead time*.
   - Describe the role of an inventory manager.
   - Analyze the elements of a good inventory management system and describe how elements relate to the organization and overall effectiveness of a dental practice.
2. Identify the types of supplies, products, and equipment that are commonly purchased for a dental practice.
3. Discuss the selection and ordering process of supplies, products, and equipment, including:
   - Compare the advantages and disadvantages of catalog ordering and supply house services and explain when it is appropriate to use the two services.
   - List the information that should be considered before an order is placed for supplies and products.
   - Explain how shipments should be received and proper storage techniques.
4. Explain the role of the Occupational Safety and Health Administration (OSHA). Describe the various sections of an effective hazard communication program and discuss what information is important to an inventory manager.

INTRODUCTION

Ordering and managing supplies in a dental practice requires organization, communication, and the cooperation of the entire dental healthcare team. Inventory control is not limited to supplies in the clinical area. Those in the laboratory and business office must also be managed. Because the financial health of the dental practice depends on controlling costs, it is necessary to establish and maintain an inventory management system (IMS) that is cost effective, efficient, and easy to manage. Having the proper supplies on hand at all times is necessary in order to offer patients the best possible care.

EXERCISES

1. List the key functions of an inventory management system.

_____

_____

_____

_____

_____

_____

_____

_____

2. List five characteristics of an inventory manager and write a brief statement about the one characteristic that you feel is key to the success of an IMS.

_____

_____

_____

_____

_____

3. Define *rate of use*.

_____

_____

4. Define *lead time*.

_____

_____

5. Define *back order*.

_____

_____

6. A good inventory management system involves seven elements. List two elements and describe how they relate to the organization of an effective dental practice.

_____

_____

_____

_____

Use the Safety Data Sheet (SDS) for Clorox® Ready-Use Bleach Pre-Diluted Cleaner – Fresh Meadow provided at the end of this chapter to answer the following questions.

7. What is the recommended use of this product?

_____

8. What is the emergency telephone number?

_____

Chapter **12** **Inventory Management**

9. Describe the odor of the product.

_____

10. What are the most important symptoms and effects of this product?

_____

11. What first aid measures would you perform if you were exposed to the condition listed in the previous question?

_____

_____

_____

_____

12. How would you safely handle this product?

_____

_____

13. What is the name of the chemical and common name of this product?

_____

14. What products and chemicals are identified in the SDS that will create a chemical reaction with Clorox® Ready-Use-Bleach Pre-Diluted Cleaner?

_____

_____

15. Describe the chemical reaction created when Clorox® Ready-Use-Bleach Pre-Diluted Cleaner reacts with one of the products listed in the SDS.

_____

_____

SAFETY DATA SHEET

Issuing Date January 5, 2015   **Revision Date** New   **Revision Number** 0

1. IDENTIFICATION OF THE SUBSTANCE/PREPARATION AND OF THE COMPANY/UNDERTAKING

Product Identifier

Product Name   Clorox® Ready-Use Bleach Pre-Diluted Cleaner - Fresh Meadow

Other means of identification

Synonyms   None

Recommended use of the chemical and restrictions on use

Recommended use   Ready-to-use bleach cleaner

Uses advised against   No information available

Details of the supplier of the safety data sheet

Supplier Address
The Clorox Company
1221 Broadway
Oakland, CA 94612

Phone: 1-510-271-7000

Emergency telephone number

Emergency Phone Numbers   For Medical Emergencies call: 1-800-446-1014
                                     For Transportation Emergencies, call Chemtrec: 1-800-424-9300

Clorox® Ready-Use Bleach Pre-Diluted Cleaner - Fresh Meadow   **Revision Date** New

2. HAZARDS IDENTIFICATION

Classification

This product is not considered hazardous by the 2012 OSHA Hazard Communication Standard (29 CFR 1910.1200).

GHS Label elements, including precautionary statements

Emergency Overview

This product is not considered hazardous by the 2012 OSHA Hazard Communication Standard (29 CFR 1910.1200).

Appearance Clear, colorless   **Physical State** Thin liquid   **Odor** Fruity, floral, bleach

Precautionary Statements - Prevention
None

Precautionary Statements - Response
None

Precautionary Statements - Storage
None

Precautionary Statements - Disposal
None

Hazards not otherwise classified (HNOC)
Not applicable

Unknown Toxicity
0.065% of the mixture consists of ingredient(s) of unknown toxicity

Other Information
No information available

Interactions with Other Chemicals
Reacts with toilet bowl cleaners, rust removers, vinegar, acids, or products containing ammonia to produce hazardous gases, such as chlorine and other chlorinated compounds.

3. COMPOSITION/INFORMATION ON INGREDIENTS

This product contains no substances that at their given concentrations are considered to be hazardous to health.

4. FIRST AID MEASURES

First aid measures

General Advice Show this safety data sheet to the doctor in attendance.

Eye Contact Hold eye open and rinse slowly and gently with water for 15–20 minutes. If present, remove contact lenses after the first 5 minutes of rinsing, then continue rinsing eye. Call a poison control center or doctor for further treatment advice.

Skin Contact Rinse skin with plenty of water. If irritation persists, call a doctor.

Inhalation Move to fresh air. If breathing problems develop, call a doctor.

Ingestion Drink a glassful of water. Call a doctor or poison control center.

Most Important symptoms and effects, both acute and delayed

Most Important Symptoms and Effects May cause eye irritation.

Indication of any immediate medical attention and special treatment needed

Notes to Physician Treat symptomatically.

5. FIRE-FIGHTING MEASURES

Suitable Extinguishing Media
Use extinguishing measures that are appropriate to local circumstances and the surrounding environment.

Unsuitable Extinguishing Media
CAUTION: Use of water spray when fighting fire may be inefficient.

Specific Hazards Arising from the Chemical

Hazardous Combustion Products
Oxides of carbon.

Explosion Data

Sensitivity to Mechanical Impact No.

Sensitivity to Static Discharge No.

Protective equipment and precautions for firefighters
As in any fire, wear self-contained breathing apparatus pressure-demand, MSHA/NIOSH (approved or equivalent) and full protective gear.

6. ACCIDENTAL RELEASE MEASURES

Personal precautions, protective equipment and emergency procedures

Personal Precautions Avoid contact with eyes.

Other Information Refer to protective measures listed in Sections 7 and 8.

Environmental precautions

Environmental Precautions See Section 12 for additional ecological information.

Methods and material for containment and cleaning up

Methods for Containment Prevent further leakage or spillage if safe to do so.

Methods for Cleaning Up Absorb and containerize. Wash residual down to sanitary sewer. Contact the sanitary treatment facility in advance to assure ability to process washed-down material.

7. HANDLING AND STORAGE

Precautions for safe handling

Handling Handle in accordance with good industrial hygiene and safety practice. Avoid contact with eyes, skin, and clothing. Do not eat, drink, or smoke when using this product.

Conditions for safe storage, including any incompatibilities

Storage Keep containers tightly closed in a dry, cool, and well-ventilated place.

Incompatible Products Toilet bowl cleaners, rust removers, vinegar, acids, and products containing ammonia.

8. EXPOSURE CONTROLS/PERSONAL PROTECTION

Control parameters

Exposure Guidelines This product does not contain any ingredients with occupational exposure limits that are at concentrations below their cut-off values/concentrations and that contribute to the hazard classification of the product.

Appropriate engineering controls

Engineering Measures Showers
Eyewash stations
Ventilation systems

Individual protection measures, such as personal protective equipment

Eye/Face Protection No special protective equipment required.

Skin and Body Protection No special protective equipment required.

Respiratory Protection No protective equipment is needed under normal use conditions. If irritation is experienced, ventilation and evacuation may be required.

Hygiene Measures Handle in accordance with good industrial hygiene and safety practice.

9. PHYSICAL AND CHEMICAL PROPERTIES

Physical and Chemical Properties

Physical State	Thin liquid
Appearance	Clear
Color	Colorless

| Odor | Fruity, floral, bleach |
| Odor Threshold | No information available |

Property	Values	Remarks/ Method
pH	12 - 12.7	None known
Melting/freezing point	No data available	None known
Boiling point / boiling range	No data available	None known
Flash Point	No data available	None known
Evaporation rate	No data available	None known
Flammability (solid, gas)	No data available	None known
Flammability Limits in Air		
Upper flammability limit	No data available	None known
Lower flammability limit	No data available	None known
Vapor pressure	No data available	None known
Vapor density	No data available	None known
Specific Gravity	~1.0	None known
Water Solubility	Complete	None known
Solubility in other solvents	No data available	None known
Partition coefficient: n-octanol/water	No data available	None known
Autoignition temperature	No data available	None known
Decomposition temperature	No data available	None known
Kinematic viscosity	No data available	None known
Dynamic viscosity	No data available	None known
Explosive Properties	Not explosive	
Oxidizing Properties	No data available	

Other Information

Softening Point	No data available
VOC Content (%)	No data available
Particle Size	No data available
Particle Size Distribution	No data available

10. STABILITY AND REACTIVITY

Reactivity
Reacts with toilet bowl cleaners, rust removers, vinegar, acids, or products containing ammonia to produce hazardous gases, such as chlorine and other chlorinated compounds.

Chemical stability
Stable under recommended storage conditions.

Possibility of Hazardous Reactions
None under normal processing.

Conditions to avoid
None known based on information supplied.

Incompatible materials
Toilet bowl cleaners, rust removers, vinegar, acids, and products containing ammonia.

Hazardous Decomposition Products
None known based on information supplied.

---

11. TOXICOLOGICAL INFORMATION

Information on likely routes of exposure

Product Information

Inhalation	Exposure to vapor or mist may irritate respiratory tract.
Eye Contact	May cause irritation.
Skin Contact	May cause slight irritation.
Ingestion	Ingestion may cause slight irritation to mucous membranes and gastrointestinal tract.

Component Information

Chemical Name	LD50 Oral	LD50 Dermal	LC50 Inhalation
Sodium hypochlorite 7681-52-9	8200 mg/kg (Rat)	>10000 mg/kg (Rabbit)	-

Information or toxicological effects

| Symptoms | Liquid may cause redness and tearing of eyes. |

Delayed and immediate effects as well as chronic effects from short and long-term exposure

Sensitization	No information available.
Mutagenic Effects	No information available.
Carcinogenicity	The table below indicates whether each agency has listed any ingredient as a carcinogen.

Chemical Name	ACGIH	IARC	NTP	OSHA
Sodium hypochlorite 7681-52-9		Group 3	-	-

IARC (International Agency for Research on Cancer)
Group 3 - Not Classifiable as to Carcinogenicity in Humans

Reproductive Toxicity	No information available.
STOT - single exposure	No information available.
STOT - repeated exposure	No information available.
Chronic Toxicity	No known effect based on information supplied.
Target Organ Effects	Respiratory system, eyes, skin, gastrointestinal tract (GI).
Aspiration Hazard	No information available.

Numerical measures of toxicity - Product Information

The following values are calculated based on chapter 3.1 of the GHS document
No information available

Clorox® Ready-Use Bleach Pre-Diluted Cleaner - Fresh Meadow

Revision Date   New

12. ECOLOGICAL INFORMATION

Ecotoxicity
No information available.

Persistence and Degradability
No information available.

Bioaccumulation
No information available.

Other adverse effects
No information available.

13. DISPOSAL CONSIDERATIONS

Disposal methods
Dispose of in accordance with all applicable federal, state, and local regulations.

Contaminated Packaging
Do not reuse empty containers.   Dispose of in accordance with all applicable federal, state, and local regulations.

14. TRANSPORT INFORMATION

DOT   Not regulated.

TDG   Not regulated.

ICAO   Not regulated.

IATA   Not regulated.

IMDG/IMO   Not regulated.

15. REGULATORY INFORMATION

Chemical Inventories

TSCA   All components of this product are either on the TSCA 8(b) Inventory or otherwise exempt from listing.

DSL/NDSL   All components are on the DSL or NDSL.

TSCA - United States Toxic Substances Control Act Section 8(b) Inventory
DSL/NDSL - Canadian Domestic Substances List/Non-Domestic Substances List

U.S. Federal Regulations

SARA 313
Section 313 of Title III of the Superfund Amendments and Reauthorization Act of 1986 (SARA).   This product does not contain any chemicals which are subject to the reporting requirements of the Act and Title 40 of the Code of Federal Regulations, Part 372

Clorox® Ready-Use Bleach Pre-Diluted Cleaner - Fresh Meadow

Revision Date   New

SARA 311/312 Hazard Categories

Acute Health Hazard	No
Chronic Health Hazard	No
Fire Hazard	No
Sudden Release of Pressure Hazard	No
Reactive Hazard	No

CWA (Clean Water Act)
This product contains the following substances which are regulated pollutants pursuant to the Clean Water Act (40 CFR 122.21 and 40 CFR 122.42)

Chemical Name	CWA - Reportable Quantities	CWA - Toxic Pollutants	CWA - Priority Pollutants	CWA - Hazardous Substances
Sodium hypochlorite 7681-52-9	100 lb			X
Sodium hydroxide 1310-73-2	1000 lb			X

CERCLA
This material, as supplied, contains one or more substances regulated as a hazardous substance under the Comprehensive Environmental Response Compensation and Liability Act (CERCLA) (40 CFR 302)

Chemical Name	Hazardous Substances RQs	Extremely Hazardous Substances RQs	RQ
Sodium hypochlorite 7681-52-9	100 lb		RQ 100 lb final RQ RQ 45.4 kg final RQ
Sodium hydroxide 1310-73-2	1000 lb	-	RQ 1000 lb final RQ RQ 454 kg final RQ

US State Regulations

California Proposition 65
This product does not contain any Proposition 65 chemicals.

U.S. State Right-to-Know Regulations

Chemical Name	New Jersey	Massachusetts	Pennsylvania	Rhode Island	Illinois
Sodium hypochlorite 7681-52-9	X	X	X	X	
Sodium hydroxide 1310-73-2	X	X	X	X	

International Regulations

Canada
WHMIS Hazard Class
Non-controlled

Clorox® Ready-Use Bleach Pre-Diluted Cleaner - Fresh Meadow

Revision Date   New

16. OTHER INFORMATION

NFPA	Health Hazard 1	Flammability 0	Instability 0	Physical and Chemical Hazards -
HMIS	Health Hazard 1	Flammability 0	Physical Hazard 0	Personal Protection -

Prepared By   Product Stewardship
23 British American Blvd.
Latham, NY 12110
1-800-572-6501

Preparation/Revision Date   January 5, 2015

Revision Note   New

Reference   1062234/169160.001

General Disclaimer
The information provided in this Safety Data Sheet is correct to the best of our knowledge, information, and belief at the date of its publication.   The information given is designed only as a guidance for safe handling, use, processing, storage, transportation, disposal, and release and is not to be considered a warranty or quality specification.   The information relates only to the specific material designated and may not be valid for such material used in combination with any other materials or in any process, unless specified in the text.

©2017 The Clorox Company. Reprinted with permission.

DENTAL PRACTICE PROCEDURAL MANUAL PROJECT (OPTIONAL)

Continue working on your Dental Practice Procedural Manual (see Workbook Chapter 6 for details).
  Suggested activities:

- Team meeting

- Review timeline

- Review Group research and writing assignments

- Complete research and writing assignments for this chapter

- Review and revise completed sections of the manual

- Individual journal entries

13 Office Equipment

LEARNING OBJECTIVES

1. List the components of a dental practice information system and explain the function of each component.
2. Describe the features and functions of a telecommunication system and explain how they can be used in a modern dental practice.
3. Compare electronic and manual systems of intraoffice communications.
4. Identify office machines commonly found in a dental practice.
5. Describe an ideal business office environment and design an ergonomic workstation. Identify important elements and state their purpose.

INTRODUCTION

Business office equipment provides the tools and resources necessary to organize tasks and integrate many different functions into a seamless flow. A computer can perform many tasks using information that is maintained in a database with speed and accuracy. A telephone system integrated with a practice management software system can identify the patient and upload his or her information before the phone is answered. Cloud computing connects many devices together, from anywhere that there are Internet connections. Business office equipment is selected according to the needs of the staff and the dental practice. Equipment can be divided into two broad categories: equipment used to gather, transfer, and store information and equipment used to create a working environment that is safe, organized, and functional.

EXERCISES

1. List and define the components of a dental practice information system.

_____

_____

_____

_____

_____

2. List and briefly describe the features of a telephone system.

_____

_____

_____

_____

_____

_____

_____

_____

_____

3. List the functions of a telecommunication system and describe how it can be used in a dental practice.

_____

_____

_____

_____

4. List seven factors to consider when setting up an ergonomic workstation.

_____

_____

_____

_____

_____

_____

5. Match the following terms to their definitions:

a. _____ Peripheral device used to activate commands   A. CPU

b. _____ Similar to a television screen   B. Keyboard

c. _____ Information needed for the computer to be able to function   C. Mouse

d. _____ Used to back up information   D. Scanner

e. _____ Main operating component of hardware   E. Modem

f. _____ Digitizes information from a document   F. Monitor

g. _____ Produces a hard copy of information   G. Printer

h. _____ Most common input device   H. Storage device

i. _____ Transfers information   I. Operating system

6. Define *intraoffice communications*.

_____

7. List the different types of intraoffice communication systems.

_____

_____

_____

_____

_____

_____

_____

8. List the types of office machines found in a dental practice.

_____

_____

_____

_____

Define the following terms:

9. Ergonomics _____

10. Background noise _____

11. Lighting _____

WHAT WOULD YOU DO?

Ergonomic Problem Solving

12. Sally, the administrative dental assistant, is complaining of lower back pain. What should she check on her chair to rectify this problem?

_____

_____

_____

_____

13. Kevin, the business manager, is complaining of eyestrain. What can he do with his video display terminal to help alleviate the strain?

_____

_____

_____

_____

_____

_____

14. Hope, the insurance biller, has been given a diagnosis of carpal tunnel syndrome. What can she do with her keyboard and mouse to help reduce the strain?

_____

_____

_____

_____

_____

_____

DENTAL PRACTICE PROCEDURAL MANUAL PROJECT (OPTIONAL)

Continue working on your Dental Practice Procedural Manual (see Workbook Chapter 6 for details).
   Suggested activities:

- Team meeting

- Review timeline

- Review Group research and writing assignments

- Complete research and writing assignments for this chapter

- Review and revise completed sections of the manual

- Individual journal entries

14 Financial Arrangement and Collection Procedures

LEARNING OBJECTIVES

1. List the elements of a financial policy and discuss the qualifying factors for each of the elements.
2. Describe the different types of financial policies and explain how they can be applied in a dental practice and how they should be communicated to the patient.
3. State the purpose of managing accounts receivable, including:
   - Explain the role of the administrative dental assistant in managing accounts receivable.
   - Interpret aging reports.
   - Classify the five levels of the collection process.
   - Place a telephone collection call.
   - Process a collection letter.
   - Implement proper collection procedures.

INTRODUCTION

The responsibility for collecting fees is shared by all members of the dental healthcare team. The team will establish the policies and then follow them. The administrative dental assistant has the most visible task. After a treatment plan has been drawn up, the administrative dental assistant will write the financial plan, present the plan to the patient, and then monitor compliance with the plan. If the plan is not followed, it is usually the administrative dental assistant who initiates collection procedures.

EXERCISES

1. Match the payment plan to its definition.

   a. _____ Payment is spread out over time

   b. _____ Payment is paid by third-party carrier

   c. _____ Payment installments are paid directly to the dental practice

   d. _____ Payment is divided by length of treatment

   e. _____ Another form of payment in full. Payment amount will be discounted and deposited directly into the practice's account

   f. _____ Payment is made immediately after dental visit by patient

   g. _____ Payment installments directed by a loan company

   A. Insurance billing

   B. Payment in full

   C. Outside payment plan

   D. In-house payment plan

   E. Extended payment plan

   F. Divided payment plan

   G. Credit card

   H. Creative payment plan

2. List the six steps to be followed in placing a telephone collection call.

_____

_____

_____

_____

_____

_____

3. At what level in the collection process should a letter be written?

   a. Level one

   b. Level two

   c. Level three

   d. Level four

   e. Level five

4. List at least two requirements of a properly written collection letter.

   _____

   _____

5. Match the following time intervals with the level of the collection process.

   a. _____ 0-30 days   A. Telephone reminder

   b. _____ 30-60 days   B. Ultimatum

   c. _____ 60-90 days   C. Mailed reminder

   d. _____ 90-120 days   D. Statement

   e. _____ Longer than 120 days   E. Collection letter

   f. _____ No response to letter   F. Turning of account over to collection

                                                 G. Friendly reminder

ACTIVITY EXERCISES

Use information located on the Treatment Plan for each of the following patients to complete a Financial Arrangement Form (located at the back of the workbook).

Jana Rogers   Angelica Green
Holly Barry   Lynn Bacca

Jana Rogers

Jana's parents both have dental insurance. After their combined benefits are calculated, it has been determined that the total benefits paid will be $1200.00.

As the administrative dental assistant, you propose the following financial arrangements.

Initial payment $75.00

Insurance estimated payment $1200.00

The balance is to be paid in three monthly payments.

Use the completed Financial Arrangement forms to answer the following questions.

6. What is the total estimate of treatment?　$_____

7. What is the balance of the estimate due?　$_____

8. What is the monthly payment?　$_____

Angelica Green

Angelica is covered by her husband's plan. His plan will pay 60% of the total estimate of treatment. In addition, Dr. Edwards will give Angelica a 10% professional courtesy discount on the balance after the insurance estimate. It is agreed that Angelica will pay the balance in six monthly payments.

Complete a Financial Arrangement Form for Angelica, and use the information to answer the following questions.

9. What is the total estimate of treatment?　$_____

10. What is the insurance estimate?　$_____

11. What is the amount of the discount?　$_____

12. What is the balance of the estimate due?　$_____

13. What is the monthly payment?　$_____

Holly Barry

Mrs. Barry is a senior citizen and will receive a 12% senior citizen discount. She has made arrangements to pay the balance in full (credit card) on April 12.

Complete a Financial Arrangement form for Mrs. Barry and use the information to answer the following questions.

14. What is the total estimate of treatment?　$_____

15. What is the amount of the discount?　$_____

16. What is the balance of the estimate due?　$_____

Lynn Bacca

Lynn's parents both have dental insurance. The combined payment will be 100% of the total estimate for treatment, less a $50.00 deductible.

Complete a Financial Arrangement Form for Lynn and use the information to answer the following questions.

17. What is the total estimate of treatment?　$_____

18. What is the insurance estimate?　$_____

Dentrix Learning Objectives

- Set up a payment agreement for a family.

- Attach a note to an account.

- Print a Truth in Lending Disclosure Statement and a coupon book for scheduled payments.

Getting Started

Before you begin this assignment you may find it helpful to watch the Dentrix Learning Edition Videos and the review the Dentrix User's Guide:

Dentrix Learning Edition Video

http://www.dentrix.com/le/on-demand-training
    Ledger

- Viewing and Navigating the Ledger

- Quiz

- Entering and Editing Transactions

- Quiz

User's Guide

Chapter 8: Ledger

- Setting up Financial Arrangements

- Payment Agreements

- Adding Notes to the Ledger

Dentrix Practice

Dentrix provides you the flexibility to set up two types of financial arrangements: (1) Payment Agreements and (2) Future Due Payment Plans. Payment Agreements can be used when treatment has been completed, and the balance will be paid over time. Future Due Payment Plans can be used when treatment will be completed over time and you want to charge an account monthly.

For this exercise you will be creating a Payment Agreement for Brent Crosby.

1. In the Ledger, select a member of the family for whom you want to create a payment agreement. When you select Brent you will notice that the Family Alert dialogue box appears. After reading the notice, click **OK**.

2. Click the **Billing/Payment Agreement** button. The Billing/Payment Agreement Information dialogue box appears.

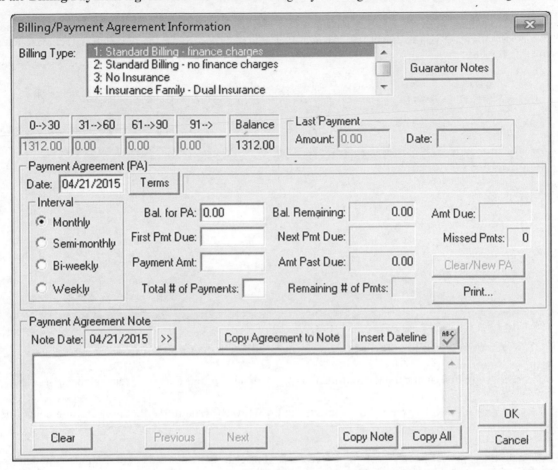

3. In the *Payment Agreement (PA)* group box, the current date appears in the Date field by default. If necessary, change the agreement date in the **Date** field.

4. Click the **Terms** button to set up the terms of the payment agreement. The Payment Agreement Terms dialogue box appears.

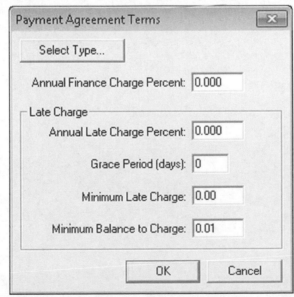

From here, terms can be set up either automatically or manually.

5. To set up the payment agreement terms automatically, click **Select Type.** The Select Payment Agreement Type dialog appears, allowing you to select the payment type you want to use for the payment agreement. Select Good Account Agreement.

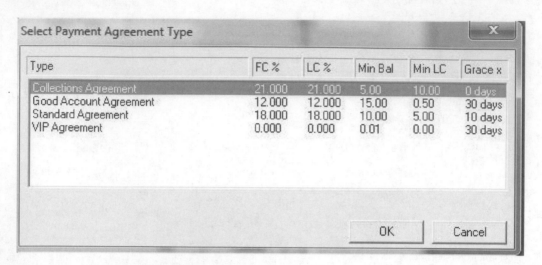

6. Click **OK** to return to the Billing/Payment Agreement Information dialog.

7. In the *Interval* group box, mark the desired interval of payments option. For this exercise check *Weekly*.

8. Enter the total amount of the agreement in the **Bal for PA** field. By default, the Learning Edition enters the patient portion of the family's balance.

9. Enter the date that the first payment is due in the **First Pmt Due field.** For this exercise enter the date one week from today.

10. Enter the payment amount or the total number of payments in the **Payment Amt** or **Total of Payments** field. For this exercise the payment will be $25.00 per week

11. To copy the agreement information click the **Copy Agreement to Note** button. Click the **Inserts Dateline** (to place today's date into the note). You can click the *ABC* button to check the spelling of the note text.

12. Click the **Print** button. The Print for Payment Agreement dialog box appear. Check the forms you would like to print. For this exercise check Truth in Lending Disclosure Statement and Coupon Book for Scheduled Payments (Plain Form)

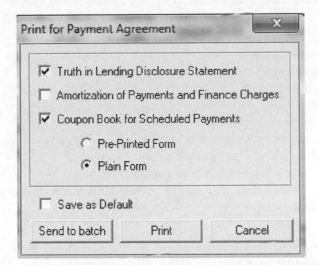

13. Click **Print**

14. Click **OK** to return to the Ledger.

Dentrix Application

Complete a Payment Agreement for Angelica Green. You will use the information given on page 82 and on the Treatment Plan you created (located in the patient's clinical record, paper and electronic.)

A. Print a Truth in Lending Disclosure Statement.

B. Print a Coupon Book for Scheduled Payments (plain paper).

DENTAL PRACTICE PROCEDURAL MANUAL PROJECT (OPTIONAL)

Continue working on your Dental Practice Procedural Manual (see Workbook Chapter 6 for details).
Suggested activities:

- Team meeting

- Review timeline

- Review Group research and writing assignments

- Complete research and writing assignments for this chapter

- Review and revise completed sections of the manual

- Individual journal entries

Chapter **14** Financial Arrangement and Collection Procedures

15 Dental Insurance Processing

LEARNING OBJECTIVES

1. Classify and identify the various types of insurance.
2. Identify the different methods of filing insurance claims and discuss the responsibility of the administrative dental assistant in filing dental claims.
3. List the types of insurance information required to determine insurance coverage.
4. Identify the two ways that insurance payments can be made and discuss payment tracking.
5. Demonstrate how to complete a dental claim form.
6. Discuss the purpose of insurance coding and differentiate between categories.
7. Describe fraudulent insurance billing, including part 5B of the American Dental Association (ADA) Code of Ethics, and identify how it applies to the administrative dental assistant.

INTRODUCTION

In the early days of dentistry, payment for dental treatment was arranged between the dentist and the patient. As dentistry progressed into a complex healthcare delivery system with a wide range of treatment options, the need for financial assistance was recognized. In the middle of the twentieth century, dental insurance was offered as a method of supplementing payment for dental treatment.

EXERCISES

1. Match each of the following descriptions of types of dental coverage with the correct term:

   a. _____ The benefits of this type of dental practice are a common name and the means for a large advertising budget.

   b. _____ Programs that dictate to patients where they can receive their dental treatment.

   c. _____ Programs in which the dental practice is paid a set amount for each patient who is enrolled in the program.

   d. _____ List of procedures covered by an insurance company and their respective dollar amounts. These fees are the same for all dentists, regardless of location.

   e. _____ Fee schedules that are calculated with distinct demographic information and criteria.

   f. _____ Designed to contain the cost of dental procedures and services by restricting the types and frequencies of procedures and services and controlling fee schedules.

   g. _____ Contract states that the dentist will use only the fee schedule preapproved by the third party. In exchange, the third party places the dentist's name on a preferred list.

   h. _____ An organization that has been legally established by a group of dentists to enter into third-party contracts.

   i. _____ Accepts responsibility for payment of dental procedures and services for members. Will not cover services if the work is done outside of the organization.

   j. _____ A method of payment that compensates the dentist according to individual services and procedures. Reimbursement is determined by established fee schedules.

   k. _____ A method of payment that bypasses an insurance company and pays directly from a fund established by an employer.

   A. Direct Reimbursement

   B. Health Maintenance Organization

   C. Individual Practice Association

   D. Managed Care

   E. Preferred Provider Organization

   F. Table of Allowances

   G. Capitation Programs

   H. Closed Panel Programs

   I. Franchise Dentistry

   J. Fee for Service

   K. UCR Plans

   L. Union Trust Funds

2. Write a short essay explaining the benefits of electronic claims processing.

3. Dental procedure codes are

    a. The same as medical procedure codes

    b. Set by each insurance company to correspond with its coverage

    c. Also known as SNODENT codes

    d. Standardized by the ADA and accepted by all third-party carriers

4. Maximum coverage can be described as

    a. The total dollar amount that will be paid for each service or procedure according to the stipulations of the insurance policy

    b. The total dollar amount that an insurance company will pay during a year

    c. The total dollar amount that an insurance company will pay for a family

    d. The total dollar amount that an insurance company will pay for a lifetime

5. The percentage of payment will vary depending on

    a. The type of procedure

    b. The insurance contract

    c. Where the patient seeks dental treatment

    d. All of the above

WHAT WOULD YOU DO?

The administrative dental assistant may be faced with many ethical and legal issues regarding the billing of insurance. In the following scenarios, use the correct reference code taken from The American Dental Association's *Principles of Ethics and Code of Professional Conduct,* Section 5B, Advisory Opinions.

6. A patient has just discovered that he will no longer be covered for insurance benefits after the end of the month. The patient is scheduled for the second week of the next month to complete his treatment plan. When you check the schedule, you discover that the dentist is taking a week off and the schedule is already overbooked. The patient asks if you can change the date to the current month so the insurance company will pay.

    a. What are your options?

    _____

    _____

    _____

    _____

    b. If you change the date, what portion of the advisory opinion addresses this issue?

    _____

111

7. The last staff meeting focused on ways to attract new patients to the dental practice. Several ideas were discussed. One of the ideas suggested that patients who have dental insurance would not be responsible for their copayment after the insurance company paid. Your assignment is to research the idea and report back to the group at the next meeting. What will you report back at the next meeting?

_____

_____

_____

_____

ACTIVITY EXERCISES

For the following exercise, you will need your clinical charts for Jana Rogers, Angelica Green, Holly Barry, and Lynn Bacca. During the exercise you will be asked to complete an insurance claim form. For this exercise use the following chart of billing codes and provider information.

Dental Insurance Coding

Procedure	Dentrix Codes*
Periodic oral evaluation	X1407
Comprehensive oral evaluation	X1437
Periapical first film	X1507
Periapical each additional film	X1510
Bitewings—four	X1567
Prophylaxis—adult	X2397
Prophylaxis—child	X2490
Topical application of fluoride—child	X2495
Sealant—per tooth	X2638
Amalgam—two-surface	X3047
Crown—porcelain fused to high noble metal	X4037
Endodontic therapy, molar	X4617
Prefabricated post and core	X5237
Periodontal scaling and root planing	X5628

*The Dentrix Codes are placeholder codes designed to mimic the style of coding used by the American Dental Association (ADA). The actual ADA codes are copyrighted in the publication *Code on Dental Procedures and Nomenclature (CDT)* and appear only with the professional version of Dentrix.

Billing Dentist Information

Use the following information to complete all claim forms (all numbers are fictitious):

Mary A. Edwards, D.D.S.
4546 North Avery Way
Canyon View, CA 91783
987-555-3210
Provider ID#34567
TIN: 95-1234568
License #10111213

8. Who is responsible for primary insurance coverage for Jana Rogers?_____

9. Who is responsible for secondary insurance coverage for Jana?_____

10. Submit a completed primary insurance claim form (claim forms are located on the following pages) for Jana. Include treatment dated 12 April, 24 April, 10 May, and 17 May.

11. Who is responsible for primary insurance coverage for Angelica Green?_____

_____

12. Identify the documentation that will be sent with Angelica's claim form._____

_____

13. Complete a claim form for Angelica for the following dates: 6 March through 24 April. Angelica has a medical condition that may contribute to periodontal disease. ICD-10, *E08.630 Diabetes due to underlying condition with periodontal disease.*

14. Who is the responsible party for Holly Barry?_____

15. What type of insurance coverage does Holly have?_____

16. Under the birthday rule, who is responsible for primary coverage for Lynn Bacca?_____

_____

17. When is the secondary insurance submitted for payment?_____

_____

18. Complete a primary insurance claim form for Lynn for 12 April and 24 April.

19. Correctly document each clinical record.

ADA American Dental Association® Dental Claim Form

HEADER INFORMATION

1. Type of Transaction (Mark all applicable boxes)

☐ Statement of Actual Services   ☐ Request for Predetermination/Preauthorization

☐ EPSDT / Title XIX

2. Predetermination/Preauthorization Number

INSURANCE COMPANY/DENTAL BENEFIT PLAN INFORMATION

3. Company/Plan Name, Address, City, State, Zip Code

OTHER COVERAGE (Mark applicable box and complete items 5-11. If none, leave blank.)

4. Dental? ☐   **Medical?** ☐   (If both, complete 5-11 for dental only.)

5. Name of Policyholder/Subscriber in #4 (Last, First, Middle Initial, Suffix)

6. Date of Birth (MM/DD/CCYY)   **7. Gender** ☐ M ☐ F   **8. Policyholder/Subscriber ID (SSN or ID#)**

9. Plan/Group Number   **10. Patient's Relationship to Person named in #5**
☐ Self ☐ Spouse ☐ Dependent ☐ Other

11. Other Insurance Company/Dental Benefit Plan Name, Address, City, State, Zip Code

POLICYHOLDER/SUBSCRIBER INFORMATION (For Insurance Company Named in #3)

12. Policyholder/Subscriber Name (Last, First, Middle Initial, Suffix), Address, City, State, Zip Code

13. Date of Birth (MM/DD/CCYY)   **14. Gender** ☐ M ☐ F   **15. Policyholder/Subscriber ID (SSN or ID#)**

16. Plan/Group Number   **17. Employer Name**

PATIENT INFORMATION

18. Relationship to Policyholder/Subscriber in #12 Above
☐ Self ☐ Spouse ☐ Dependent Child ☐ Other   **19. Reserved For Future Use**

20. Name (Last, First, Middle Initial, Suffix), Address, City, State, Zip Code

21. Date of Birth (MM/DD/CCYY)   **22. Gender** ☐ M ☐ F   **23. Patient ID/Account # (Assigned by Dentist)**

RECORD OF SERVICES PROVIDED

	24. Procedure Date (MM/DD/CCYY)	25. Area of Oral Cavity	26. Tooth System	27. Tooth Number(s) or Letter(s)	28. Tooth Surface	29. Procedure Code	29a. Diag. Pointer	29b. Qty.	30. Description	31. Fee
1										
2										
3										
4										
5										
6										
7										
8										
9										
10										

33. Missing Teeth Information   (Place an "X" on each missing tooth.)

1	2	3	4	5	6	7	8	9	10	11	12	13	14	15	16
32	31	30	29	28	27	26	25	24	23	22	21	20	19	18	17

34. Diagnosis Code List Qualifier ☐   (ICD-9 = B; ICD-10 = AB)

34a. Diagnosis Code(s)   A _____   C _____
(Primary diagnosis in "A")   B _____   D _____

31a. Other Fee(s)

32. Total Fee

35. Remarks

AUTHORIZATIONS

36. I have been informed of the treatment plan and associated fees. I agree to be responsible for all charges for dental services and materials not paid by my dental benefit plan, unless prohibited by law, or the treating dentist or dental practice has a contractual agreement with my plan prohibiting all or a portion of such charges. To the extent permitted by law, I consent to your use and disclosure of my protected health information to carry out payment activities in connection with this claim.

X _____
Patient/Guardian Signature   Date

37. I hereby authorize and direct payment of the dental benefits otherwise payable to me, directly to the below named dentist or dental entity.

X _____
Subscriber Signature   Date

BILLING DENTIST OR DENTAL ENTITY (Leave blank if dentist or dental entity is not submitting claim on behalf of the patient or insured/subscriber.)

48. Name, Address, City, State, Zip Code

49. NPI   **50. License Number**   **51. SSN or TIN**

52. Phone Number ( ) -   **52a. Additional Provider ID**

ANCILLARY CLAIM/TREATMENT INFORMATION

38. Place of Treatment ☐ (e.g. 11=office; 22=O/P Hospital)
(Use "Place of Service Codes for Professional Claims")

39. Enclosures (Y or N) ☐

40. Is Treatment for Orthodontics?
☐ No (Skip 41-42)   ☐ Yes (Complete 41-42)

41. Date Appliance Placed (MM/DD/CCYY)

42. Months of Treatment   **43. Replacement of Prosthesis** ☐ No ☐ Yes (Complete 44)   **44. Date of Prior Placement (MM/DD/CCYY)**

45. Treatment Resulting from
☐ Occupational illness/injury   ☐ Auto accident   ☐ Other accident

46. Date of Accident (MM/DD/CCYY)   **47. Auto Accident State**

TREATING DENTIST AND TREATMENT LOCATION INFORMATION

53. I hereby certify that the procedures as indicated by date are in progress (for procedures that require multiple visits) or have been completed.

X _____
Signed (Treating Dentist)   Date

54. NPI   **55. License Number**

56. Address, City, State, Zip Code   **56a. Provider Specialty Code**

57. Phone Number ( ) -   **58. Additional Provider ID**

To reorder call 800.947.4746
or go online at adacatalog.org

The American Dental Association dental claim form. (Copyright © 2012 American Dental Association, Chicago, Ill.)

ADA American Dental Association® Dental Claim Form

HEADER INFORMATION

1. Type of Transaction (Mark all applicable boxes)

☐ Statement of Actual Services   ☐ Request for Predetermination/Preauthorization

☐ EPSDT / Title XIX

2. Predetermination/Preauthorization Number

INSURANCE COMPANY/DENTAL BENEFIT PLAN INFORMATION

3. Company/Plan Name, Address, City, State, Zip Code

OTHER COVERAGE (Mark applicable box and complete items 5-11. If none, leave blank.)

4. Dental? ☐   Medical? ☐   (If both, complete 5-11 for dental only.)

5. Name of Policyholder/Subscriber in #4 (Last, First, Middle Initial, Suffix)

6. Date of Birth (MM/DD/CCYY)   7. Gender ☐ M ☐ F   8. Policyholder/Subscriber ID (SSN or ID#)

9. Plan/Group Number   10. Patient's Relationship to Person named in #5
☐ Self ☐ Spouse ☐ Dependent ☐ Other

11. Other Insurance Company/Dental Benefit Plan Name, Address, City, State, Zip Code

POLICYHOLDER/SUBSCRIBER INFORMATION (For Insurance Company Named in #3)

12. Policyholder/Subscriber Name (Last, First, Middle Initial, Suffix), Address, City, State, Zip Code

13. Date of Birth (MM/DD/CCYY)   14. Gender ☐ M ☐ F   15. Policyholder/Subscriber ID (SSN or ID#)

16. Plan/Group Number   17. Employer Name

PATIENT INFORMATION

18. Relationship to Policyholder/Subscriber in #12 Above
☐ Self ☐ Spouse ☐ Dependent Child ☐ Other

19. Reserved For Future Use

20. Name (Last, First, Middle Initial, Suffix), Address, City, State, Zip Code

21. Date of Birth (MM/DD/CCYY)   22. Gender ☐ M ☐ F   23. Patient ID/Account # (Assigned by Dentist)

RECORD OF SERVICES PROVIDED

	24. Procedure Date (MM/DD/CCYY)	25. Area of Oral Cavity	26. Tooth System	27. Tooth Number(s) or Letter(s)	28. Tooth Surface	29. Procedure Code	29a. Diag. Pointer	29b. Qty.	30. Description	31. Fee
1										
2										
3										
4										
5										
6										
7										
8										
9										
10										

33. Missing Teeth Information (Place an "X" on each missing tooth.)

1 2 3 4 5 6 7 8 9 10 11 12 13 14 15 16

32 31 30 29 28 27 26 25 24 23 22 21 20 19 18 17

34. Diagnosis Code List Qualifier ☐ (ICD-9 = B; ICD-10 = AR)

34a. Diagnosis Code(s)   A _____   C _____

(Primary diagnosis in "A")   B _____   D _____

31a. Other Fee(s)

32. Total Fee

35. Remarks

AUTHORIZATIONS

36. I have been informed of the treatment plan and associated fees. I agree to be responsible for all charges for dental services and materials not paid by my dental benefit plan, unless prohibited by law, or the treating dentist or dental practice has a contractual agreement with my plan prohibiting all or a portion of such charges. To the extent permitted by law, I consent to your use and disclosure of my protected health information to carry out payment activities in connection with this claim

X_____
Patient/Guardian Signature   Date

37. I hereby authorize and direct payment of the dental benefits otherwise payable to me, directly to the below named dentist or dental entity.

X_____
Subscriber Signature   Date

BILLING DENTIST OR DENTAL ENTITY (Leave blank if dentist or dental entity is not submitting claim on behalf of the patient or insured/subscriber.)

48. Name, Address, City, State, Zip Code

49. NPI   50. License Number   51. SSN or TIN

52. Phone Number ( ) -   52a. Additional Provider ID

ANCILLARY CLAIM/TREATMENT INFORMATION

38. Place of Treatment ☐ (e.g. 11=office; 22=O/P Hospital)
(Use "Place of Service Codes for Professional Claims")

39. Enclosures (Y or N) ☐

40. Is Treatment for Orthodontics?
☐ No (Skip 41-42) ☐ Yes (Complete 41-42)

41. Date Appliance Placed (MM/DD/CCYY)

42. Months of Treatment   43. Replacement of Prosthesis ☐ No ☐ Yes (Complete 44)   44. Date of Prior Placement (MM/DD/CCYY)

45. Treatment Resulting from
☐ Occupational illness/injury ☐ Auto accident ☐ Other accident

46. Date of Accident (MM/DD/CCYY)   47. Auto Accident State

TREATING DENTIST AND TREATMENT LOCATION INFORMATION

53. I hereby certify that the procedures as indicated by date are in progress (for procedures that require multiple visits) or have been completed.

X_____
Signed (Treating Dentist)   Date

54. NPI   55. License Number

56. Address, City, State, Zip Code   56a. Provider Specialty Code

57. Phone Number ( ) -   58. Additional Provider ID

©2012 American Dental Association
J430D (Same as ADA Dental Claim Form – J430, J431, J432, J433, J434)

To reorder call 800.947.4746
or go online at adacatalog.org

The American Dental Association dental claim form. (Copyright © 2012 American Dental Association, Chicago, Ill.)

115

ADA American Dental Association® Dental Claim Form

HEADER INFORMATION

1. Type of Transaction (Mark all applicable boxes)

☐ Statement of Actual Services ☐ Request for Predetermination/Preauthorization

☐ EPSDT / Title XIX

2. Predetermination/Preauthorization Number

INSURANCE COMPANY/DENTAL BENEFIT PLAN INFORMATION

3. Company/Plan Name, Address, City, State, Zip Code

OTHER COVERAGE (Mark applicable box and complete items 5-11. If none, leave blank.)

4. Dental? ☐   **Medical?** ☐   (If both, complete 5-11 for dental only.)

5. Name of Policyholder/Subscriber in #4 (Last, First, Middle Initial, Suffix)

6. Date of Birth (MM/DD/CCYY)   **7. Gender** ☐ M ☐ F   **8. Policyholder/Subscriber ID (SSN or ID#)**

9. Plan/Group Number   **10. Patient's Relationship to Person named in #5** ☐ Self ☐ Spouse ☐ Dependent ☐ Other

11. Other Insurance Company/Dental Benefit Plan Name, Address, City, State, Zip Code

POLICYHOLDER/SUBSCRIBER INFORMATION (For Insurance Company Named in #3)

12. Policyholder/Subscriber Name (Last, First, Middle Initial, Suffix), Address, City, State, Zip Code

13. Date of Birth (MM/DD/CCYY)   **14. Gender** ☐ M ☐ F   **15. Policyholder/Subscriber ID (SSN or ID#)**

16. Plan/Group Number   **17. Employer Name**

PATIENT INFORMATION

18. Relationship to Policyholder/Subscriber in #12 Above ☐ Self ☐ Spouse ☐ Dependent Child ☐ Other   **19. Reserved For Future Use**

20. Name (Last, First, Middle Initial, Suffix), Address, City, State, Zip Code

21. Date of Birth (MM/DD/CCYY)   **22. Gender** ☐ M ☐ F   **23. Patient ID/Account # (Assigned by Dentist)**

RECORD OF SERVICES PROVIDED

	24. Procedure Date (MM/DD/CCYY)	25. Area of Oral Cavity	26. Tooth System	27. Tooth Number(s) or Letter(s)	28. Tooth Surface	29. Procedure Code	29a. Diag. Pointer	29b. Qty.	30. Description	31. Fee
1										
2										
3										
4										
5										
6										
7										
8										
9										
10										

33. Missing Teeth Information (Place an "X" on each missing tooth.)

| 1 | 2 | 3 | 4 | 5 | 6 | 7 | 8 | 9 | 10 | 11 | 12 | 13 | 14 | 15 | 16 |
| 32 | 31 | 30 | 29 | 28 | 27 | 26 | 25 | 24 | 23 | 22 | 21 | 20 | 19 | 18 | 17 |

34. Diagnosis Code List Qualifier (ICD-9 = B; ICD-10 = AB)

34a. Diagnosis Code(s) A _____ C _____
(Primary diagnosis in "**A**") B _____ D _____

31a. Other Fee(s)

32. Total Fee

35. Remarks

AUTHORIZATIONS

36. I have been informed of the treatment plan and associated fees. I agree to be responsible for all charges for dental services and materials not paid by my dental benefit plan, unless prohibited by law, or the treating dentist or dental practice has a contractual agreement with my plan prohibiting all or a portion of such charges. To the extent permitted by law, I consent to your use and disclosure of my protected health information to carry out payment activities in connection with this claim.

X _____
Patient/Guardian Signature   Date

37. I hereby authorize and direct payment of the dental benefits otherwise payable to me, directly to the below named dentist or dental entity.

X _____
Subscriber Signature   Date

BILLING DENTIST OR DENTAL ENTITY (Leave blank if dentist or dental entity is not submitting claim on behalf of the patient or insured/subscriber.)

48. Name, Address, City, State, Zip Code

49. NPI   **50. License Number**   **51. SSN or TIN**

52. Phone Number ( ) -   **52a. Additional Provider ID**

ANCILLARY CLAIM/TREATMENT INFORMATION

38. Place of Treatment _____ (e.g. 11=office; 22=O/P Hospital)
(Use "Place of Service Codes for Professional Claims")

39. Enclosures (Y or N) ☐

40. Is Treatment for Orthodontics? ☐ No (Skip 41-42) ☐ Yes (Complete 41-42)

41. Date Appliance Placed (MM/DD/CCYY)

42. Months of Treatment   **43. Replacement of Prosthesis** ☐ No ☐ Yes (Complete 44)   **44. Date of Prior Placement (MM/DD/CCYY)**

45. Treatment Resulting from ☐ Occupational illness/injury ☐ Auto accident ☐ Other accident

46. Date of Accident (MM/DD/CCYY)   **47. Auto Accident State**

TREATING DENTIST AND TREATMENT LOCATION INFORMATION

53. I hereby certify that the procedures as indicated by date are in progress (for procedures that require multiple visits) or have been completed.

X _____
Signed (Treating Dentist)   Date

54. NPI   **55. License Number**

56. Address, City, State, Zip Code   **56a. Provider Specialty Code**

57. Phone Number ( ) -   **58. Additional Provider ID**

The American Dental Association dental claim form. (Copyright © 2012 American Dental Association, Chicago, Ill.)

Dentrix Learning Objectives

■ Create an insurance claim.

■ Create a pretreatment estimate.

■ Add attachments or add other required information into an insurance claim.

■ Print an insurance claim.

Getting Started

Before you begin this assignment you may find it helpful to review the Dentrix User's Guide:

Chapter 8: Ledger

   Claim Processing

   Working with Treatment Plans

Dentrix Practice

It may be necessary to create insurance claims for all procedures posted on a certain day or select only certain procedures to be included on the insurance claim. You can also create a pre-treatment estimate for procedures that require pre-determination.

Creating insurance claims

When work has been completed and is posted in the Ledger, you can create a primary insurance claim for the procedures.

1. In the Ledger select a patient. For this exercise select Mary Brown

2. Create the insurance claim.

   If the procedures for the claim were posted on another day, select the procedures and click the **Ins. Select Proc.** Button. For this exercise select all of the procedures.
   If the procedures for the claim were posted today, click the **Ins. Today's Proc** button.
   (You will use this method for the exercises in Chapter 17)
   Tip: When you have multiple procedures to include, hold the right mouse button or press the Ctrl key and click each procedure to be included on the claim with the left mouse button.

Printing an insurance claim

In the majority of dental offices claims will be batched and submitted electronically. Occasionally they may be printed. For this exercise you will print your completed insurance claim.

1. From the Ledger click File>office manager> the Batch Processor window appears. Select the claim you would like to print (Mary Brown)

2. Click File>Print. Close Batch Processor Window

Creating pre-treatment estimates

When procedures require pre-determination by the insurance carrier it will be necessary to create a *Request for Predetermination/Preauthorization* claim.

1. In the Ledger, select a patient. For this exercise select Carol Little

2. Create the pre-treatment estimate.

   If only certain treatment-planned procedures need to be included on the pre-treatment estimate, select the procedures and click the **Ins. Selected Proc.** Button. For this exercise select tooth # 19
   If all treatment-planned procedures need to be included on the pre-treatment estimate, click the **Ins. All Proc** button.

117

Adding additional information to a claim

When insurance claims require additional information such as, student status, attachments, reason for preauthorization, additional insurance information, or other information you will need to add the information to the claim.

1. In the Ledger, select a patient. For this exercise select Carol Little.

2. Double click a claim, the Primary Dental Insurance Claim window appears.

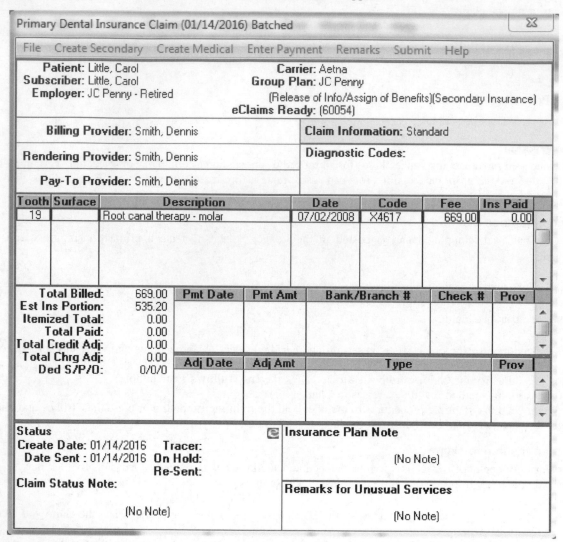

3. Double click the **Claim Information** block. The Insurance Claim Information dialog box appears.

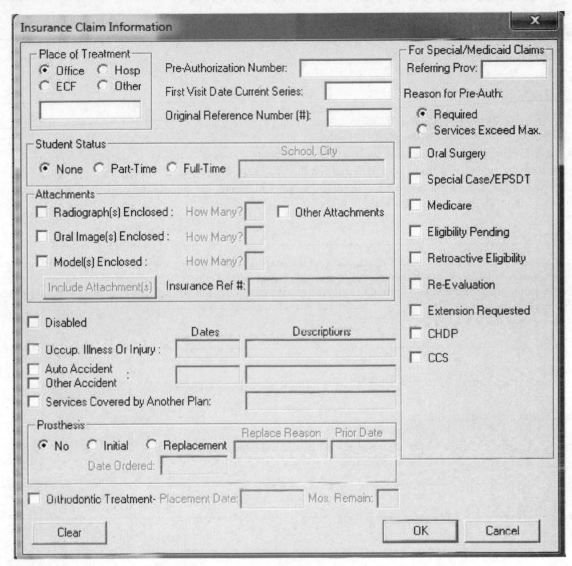

4. In the *Attachments* group box, chick the appropriate attachment option. For this exercise check Radiograph(s) 1

5. Click **OK**

6. Close the claim to return to the Ledger.

Dentrix Application

For this exercise you will create and print a Dental Pretreatment Estimate for your patient Jana Rogers for the treatment of tooth #30. Please read the section in the Dentrix *User's Guide,* Family File, entitled "Creating a Dental Pre-Treatment Estimate" and complete the following patient-related forms:

20. Print a dental pretreatment estimate for Jana Rogers for the treatment of tooth #30.

   a. What is the total estimate charge?

   b. Did you include x-rays?

   c. What is the Dentrix code used for the root canal?

   d. What is listed in box #36?

16 Bookkeeping Procedures: Accounts Payable

LEARNING OBJECTIVES

1. Describe the function of accounts payable.
2. Formulate a system to organize accounts payable.
3. Analyze the methods of check writing and state their functions.
4. Discuss steps to reconcile a bank statement and list the necessary information.
5. Discuss payroll, including the information needed for a payroll record, the calculation of payroll and necessary taxes, reporting of payroll, and payroll services.

INTRODUCTION

Accounts payable is a system by which all dental practice expenditures are organized, verified, and categorized. The system identifies when checks for bills (including payroll) are to be written, verifies charges, and categorizes expenditures. Other elements of the accounts payable system include reconciliation of the checking accounts and preparation of documents for the accountant.

EXERCISES

1. Describe the function of accounts payable.

   _____

2. List and explain the different ways a payment authorization can be made.

   _____

   _____

   _____

   _____

3. Identify the parts of a check, refer to page 237 in the text.

   a. What is the number that identifies the name of the bank and the region where it is located?

   b. What is the bank number code?

   c. What is the account number?

   d. What is the check number?

   e. Who is issuing the check?

4. List the information needed for a payroll record.

_____

_____

_____

_____

_____

_____

_____

_____

ACTIVITY EXERCISE

For the following exercises, you will be calculating payroll and writing checks.
   Scenario: Your assignment today as the administrative dental assistant is to calculate the payroll.

5. Total the hours worked for Sue Smith:

   Time Card

   Employee: Sue Smith

   Pay period: 4/1 to 4/13

Date	Time in	Time out	Time in	Time out	Total Hours
4/1	8:00	12:00	1:30	5:30	
4/2	8:15	12:00	1:00	5:00	
4/3	10:00	1:00	2:00	6:00	
4/5	7:45	12:15	1:30	5:00	
4/6	7:30	1:30			
4/9	8:00	12:00	1:30	5:30	
4/10	8:00	12:00	1:00	5:00	
4/11	10:00	1:00	2:00	6:00	
4/12	7:45	12:15	1:30	5:00	
4/13	7:30	1:30			
TOTAL HOURS WORKED					

6. Refer to Sue's payroll record (see p. 97) for the following information:
   Marital Status   _____
   Exemptions   _____
   Rate of Pay   _____

7. Calculate the following for Sue Smith:
   Gross Salary (Refer to Sue's payroll record and the time card to calculate.) $ _____
   Federal Withholding (See Tax Table on the following page.) $ _____
   FICA Tax (6.2%) $ _____
   Medicare (1.45%) $ _____
   Pension (6%) $ _____

8. Refer to Edith's payroll record (p. 97) for the following information:
   Marital Status   _____
   Exemptions   _____
   Rate of Pay   _____

9. Calculate the following for Edith Gates:
   Gross Salary (Refer to Edith's payroll record to calculate.) $ _____
   Federal Withholding (See Tax Table on the following page.) $ _____
   FICA Tax (6.2%) $ _____
   Medicare (1.45%) $ _____
   Pension (6%) $ _____

Date all checks 4/13 of the current year.

Wage Bracket Method Tables for Income Tax Withholding

MARRIED Persons—SEMIMONTHLY Payroll Period

(For Wages Paid through December 31, 2015)

And the wages are—		And the number of withholding allowances claimed is—										
At least	But less than	0	1	2	3	4	5	6	7	8	9	10
		The amount of income tax to be withheld is—										
$1,600	$1,620	$149	$124	$99	$75	$59	$42	$25	$9	$0	$0	$0
1,620	1,640	152	127	102	77	61	44	27	11	0	0	0
1,640	1,660	155	130	105	80	63	46	29	13	0	0	0
1,660	1,680	158	133	108	83	65	48	31	15	0	0	0
1,680	1,700	161	136	111	86	67	50	33	17	0	0	0
1,700	1,720	164	139	114	89	69	52	35	19	2	0	0
1,720	1,740	167	142	117	92	71	54	37	21	4	0	0
1,740	1,760	170	145	120	95	73	56	39	23	6	0	0
1,760	1,780	173	148	123	98	75	58	41	25	8	0	0
1,780	1,800	176	151	126	101	77	60	43	27	10	0	0
1,800	1,820	179	154	129	104	79	62	45	29	12	0	0
1,820	1,840	182	157	132	107	82	64	47	31	14	0	0
1,840	1,860	185	160	135	110	85	66	49	33	16	0	0
1,860	1,880	188	163	138	113	88	68	51	35	18	1	0
1,880	1,900	191	166	141	116	91	70	53	37	20	3	0
1,900	1,920	194	169	144	119	94	72	55	39	22	5	0
1,920	1,940	197	172	147	122	97	74	57	41	24	7	0
1,940	1,960	200	175	150	125	100	76	59	43	26	9	0
1,960	1,980	203	178	153	128	103	78	61	45	28	11	0
1,980	2,000	206	181	156	131	106	81	63	47	30	13	0
2,000	2,020	209	184	159	134	109	84	65	49	32	15	0
2,020	2,040	212	187	162	137	112	87	67	51	34	17	1
2,040	2,060	215	190	165	140	115	90	69	53	36	19	3
2,060	2,080	218	193	168	143	118	93	71	55	38	21	5
2,080	2,100	221	196	171	146	121	96	73	57	40	23	7
2,100	2,120	224	199	174	149	124	99	75	59	42	25	9
2,120	2,140	227	202	177	152	127	102	77	61	44	27	11
2,140	2,160	230	205	180	155	130	105	80	63	46	29	13
2,160	2,180	233	208	183	158	133	108	83	65	48	31	15
2,180	2,200	236	211	186	161	136	111	86	67	50	33	17
2,200	2,220	239	214	189	164	139	114	89	69	52	35	19
2,220	2,240	242	217	192	167	142	117	92	71	54	37	21
2,240	2,260	245	220	195	170	145	120	95	73	56	39	23
2,260	2,280	248	223	198	173	148	123	98	75	58	41	25
2,280	2,300	251	226	201	176	151	126	101	77	60	43	27
2,300	2,320	254	229	204	179	154	129	104	79	62	45	29
2,320	2,340	257	232	207	182	157	132	107	82	64	47	31
2,340	2,360	260	235	210	185	160	135	110	85	66	49	33
2,360	2,380	263	238	213	188	163	138	113	88	68	51	35
2,380	2,400	266	241	216	191	166	141	116	91	70	53	37
2,400	2,420	269	244	219	194	169	144	119	94	72	55	39
2,420	2,440	272	247	222	197	172	147	122	97	74	57	41
2,440	2,460	275	250	225	200	175	150	125	100	76	59	43
2,460	2,480	278	253	228	203	178	153	128	103	78	61	45
2,480	2,500	281	256	231	206	181	156	131	106	81	63	47
2,500	2,520	284	259	234	209	184	159	134	109	84	65	49
2,520	2,540	287	262	237	212	187	162	137	112	87	67	51
2,540	2,560	290	265	240	215	190	165	140	115	90	69	53
2,560	2,580	293	268	243	218	193	168	143	118	93	71	55
2,580	2,600	296	271	246	221	196	171	146	121	96	73	57
2,600	2,620	299	274	249	224	199	174	149	124	99	75	59
2,620	2,640	302	277	252	227	202	177	152	127	102	77	61
2,640	2,660	305	280	255	230	205	180	155	130	105	80	63
2,660	2,680	308	283	258	233	208	183	158	133	108	83	65
2,680	2,700	311	286	261	236	211	186	161	136	111	86	67
2,700	2,720	314	289	264	239	214	189	164	139	114	89	69
2,720	2,740	317	292	267	242	217	192	167	142	117	92	71
2,740	2,760	320	295	270	245	220	195	170	145	120	95	73
2,760	2,780	323	298	273	248	223	198	173	148	123	98	75
2,780	2,800	326	301	276	251	226	201	176	151	126	101	77
2,800	2,820	329	304	279	254	229	204	179	154	129	104	79
2,820	2,840	332	307	282	257	232	207	182	157	132	107	82
2,840	2,860	335	310	285	260	235	210	185	160	135	110	85
2,860	2,880	338	313	288	263	238	213	188	163	138	113	88
2,880	2,900	341	316	291	266	241	216	191	166	141	116	91
2,900	2,920	344	319	294	269	244	219	194	169	144	119	94

$2,920 and over   Use Table 3(b) for a **MARRIED person** on page 45. Also see the instructions on page 43.

Chapter **16** **Bookkeeping Procedures: Accounts Payable**

10. Using information from Question 7, complete the following payroll record for Sue Smith:

| Marital status M |
| Number of Exp 1 |

EMPLOYEE'S PAYROLL RECORD

Name: **Sue Smith**
Address: **18 N. Fox Glenn**
Telephone: **555-3816**
Occupation: **Dental Assistant**
Pay rate: **$23.50**

Social Security Number: **620-31-8752**
City: **CanyonView**   Zip code: _____
Date of birth: **06/20/70**
Date of employment: **10/2**

	Date	Check number	Gross salary	Fed W/H	FICA	M/C	State W/H	Other	Net check
	Total								

11. Write a payroll check for Ms. Smith.

Mary A. Edwards, D.D.S.
4546 North Avery Way
Canyon View, CA 91783

YOUR BANK HERE
CITY, STATE ZIP

00-0000
0000

No. 3223

PAY _____ DOLLARS

TO THE
ORDER OF _____

DISC.	DATE	CHECK NO.	AMOUNT	
			DOLLARS	CTS.

YOUR NAME HERE

⑈⑈OO₁₈54⑈⑈ ⑈:OOOOOOOOO⑈: OOOOOOOO⑈ _____

12. Using information from Question 9, complete the following payroll record for Edith Gates:

| Marital status M |
| Number of Exp 3 |

EMPLOYEE'S PAYROLL RECORD

Name: **Edith Gates**
Address: **46472 5th St.**
Telephone: **555-0182**
Occupation: **Insurance Clerk**
Pay rate: **$1800.00 Semimonthly**

Social Security Number: **608-31-8211**
City: **Canyon View**   Zip code: _____
Date of birth: **10/18/46**
Date of employment: _____

	Date	Check number	Gross salary	Fed W/H	FICA	M/C	State W/H	Other	Net check
	Total								

13. Write a payroll check for Ms. Gates.

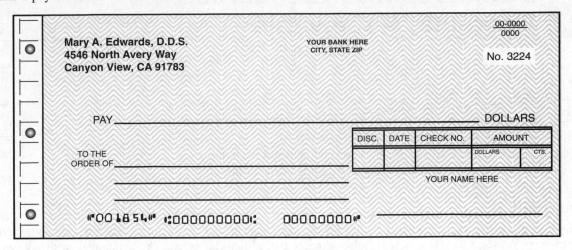

125

17 Bookkeeping Procedures: Accounts Receivable

LEARNING OBJECTIVES

1. Explain the role of the administrative dental assistant in the management of patient financial transactions.
2. Identify the components of financial records organization.
3. Perform the steps in the daily routine for managing patient transactions.
4. List and explain the types of financial reports used in a dental office.

INTRODUCTION

Dentistry, like any business, is mandated by federal and state regulations to maintain a system that documents the collection of monies. Smart business practice also requires that a financial system be maintained, with both accounts receivable and accounts payable. Accounts receivable is the system that records all financial transactions between a patient and the dental practice. This system calculates the amount of money owed to the dental practice by accounting for charges and payments. Accounts payable is the system that records all monies the dental practice owes others. It is the responsibility of the administrative dental assistant to maintain accurate records in the management of accounts receivable and accounts payable.

EXERCISES

1. Describe the routine for managing financial transactions.

_____

_____

_____

_____

_____

_____

_____

2. Explain the purpose of an audit report.

_____

_____

3. List the types of reports and identify their primary use in a dental practice.

_____

_____

_____

_____

_____

_____

_____

DENTRIX EXERCISE

As part of the daily routine you will perform a series of tasks that will organize the day, track patient treatment, post patient transactions, check out a patient, and schedule new appointments.

Before you can complete the following tasks, it will be necessary to move the patients you scheduled during the Dentrix Appointment Book Chapter 10 exercise to the current day in the appointment book. If you have not scheduled patients you can select patients from the Appointment List in the Appointments module (Appt List> Unscheduled List.).

Moving Appointments

Whether a patient needs to reschedule or the office needs to lighten the schedule, from time to time you will need to move an already scheduled appointment to a new date or time. You can either move an appointment directly to a new date and time or move it temporarily to the Pinboard. *Note:* You can move appointments in Day View and Week View but not in Month View.

Moving an appointment directly to a new date and time

1. Set the Day View or Week View, depending on whether you are moving the appointment to a different time in the same day or to a different day of the same week.

2. In Appointment Book, click the appointment that you want to move and drag it to the new date.

3. When the **Move Appointment** message appears, click **Yes.**

Moving an appointment to the Pinboard

1. In the Appointment Book, click the appointment that you want to move and drag it to the Pinboard in the upper right corner of the Appointment Book.

2. Find a new date and time for the appointment.

3. Click the appointment icon on the Pinboard and drag the appointment to the new date and time.

4. When the **Move Appointment** message appears, click **Yes.**

Tip: If you know the exact date and time to which you want to move an appointment, double-click the appointment to open the **Appointment Information** dialogue box, enter the new date and time in the date and time fields, and click **OK.**

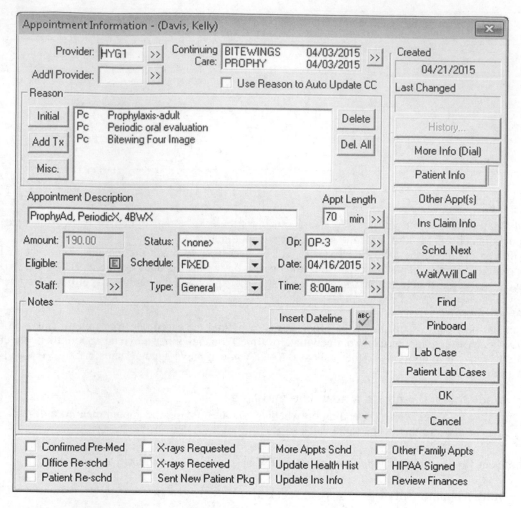

Moving an appointment from a list

1. In the Appointment Book, click Appt List and select the list you wish to use. For this exercise use the Unscheduled List.

2. Drag the patient you wish to schedule to the selected date and time in the appointment book and click **Yes.**

Route Slips

The Dentrix Route Slip can be used for a variety of information purposes: as a reminder of Medical Alerts, for patient notes, and for collection information for patients being seen that day. Also, all future appointments for every family member appear on the Patient Route Slip. To generate a route slip:

1. From the Appointment Book, select an appointment (single click).

2. From the Appointment Book toolbar, click the **Print Route Slip** button. The Print Route Slip dialogue box appears.

3. To print the report immediately, click the **Print** button.

Checking in a Patient

When a patient arrives in the dental office you will be able to change the status of the patient and alert team members that their patient has arrived and is ready to be seen. You will also need to check the patient's file for any alerts, changes in information and medical history. All of these tasks can be completed directly from the Appointment Information dialogue box.

1. Double click the selected patient in the appointment book. The Appointment Information dialogue box will appear, (see previous Appointment Information box)

   ■ In the Appointment Description group box you can change the status. *Note*: The selections in the Status box is a method used to let you or any viewer know where you are in the appointment process and is an excellent communication tool.

2. Click OK when you are finished.

Posting Scheduled Work

Once an appointment has been completed, you can quickly post procedures attached to the appointment with the click of one button. To post appointment procedures:

1. In the Appointment Book, select the Appointment you want to post as complete.

2. From the Appointment Book toolbar, click the **Set Complete** button. The Set Appointment Procedures Complete dialogue box appears.

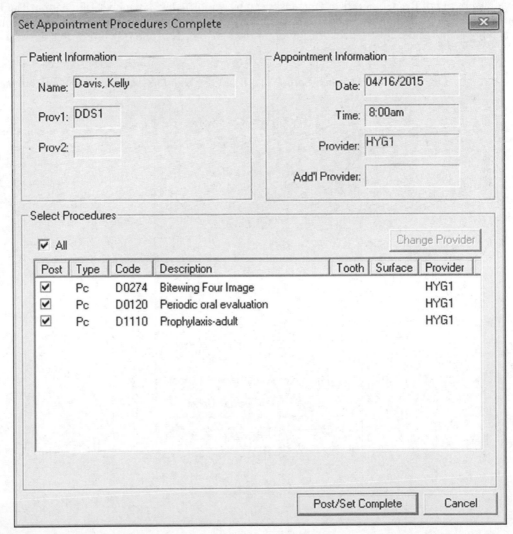

3. All procedures attached to the appointment are highlighted. If a procedure has not been completed on this visit, click it once to remove the highlight. *Note:* If the patient has had additional treatment completed during the visit, post the work in the Chart or Ledger.

4. Click the **Set Complete** button. The procedures are posted to the Chart/Ledger, and the appointment turns gray, indicating that it has been completed.

Scheduling the Next Appointment

1. Right-click on the patient in the Appointment Book (notice all of the options).

2. Click **Other Appointments.**

3. Select the treatment to be scheduled.

4. Click **Create New Appt.**

5. Complete the **Appointment Information** dialogue box. (*Reason* group box and *Appointment Description* group box, Date and Time.

6. Click **OK** (this will take you to the day and time you selected, if this is correct return to the current date.)

Fast Checkout Button

When a patient checks out of the dental office, three tasks can be completed with the click of a button. The **Fast Checkout** button, located on the Ledger toolbar, allows you to quickly post a payment, generate an insurance claim, and print a receipt. You can customize the **Fast Checkout** button to meet the needs of the office. For this exercise, set the following options:

1. Select **File** and then **Fast Checkout Options Setup.** The Fast Checkout Options Setup dialogue box appears.

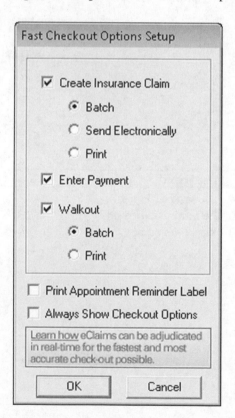

2. Set up the following tasks:

    a. Click **Create Insurance Claim;** then select **Print.**

    b. Click **Enter Payment.**

    c. Click **Walkout,** and then select **Print.**

    d. Click **Always Show Checkout options.**

    e. Click **OK.**

Using fast checkout

1. Right click the selected patient. Click **Ledger**.

2. If you have not already posted the procedures for this patient, post them at this time.

3. From the Ledger toolbar, click the **Fast Checkout** button. If you have set the button option to always show Checkout Options, the Checkout Options Setup dialogue box appears.

4. Select the desired option(s) if necessary.

5. Click **OK.**

6. The Enter Payment dialogue box appears. Enter the payment information and click **OK.**

End of Day Tasks

At the end of each day you will need to complete all posting of daily transactions, prepare a bank deposit, generate a Day Sheet Report, complete insurance processing and account for all transactions.

Generate a day sheet report

The Day Sheet shows all transactions entered in your database for a given date range. To generate a Day sheet:

1. In the Office Manager, select **Reports>Management>Day Sheets (Charges and Receipts)** or click the Day Sheet Report button. The Day Sheet dialog box appears.

2. In the *Select Provider* group box, select the desired provider range. For this exercise select all.

3. In the *Select Billing Type* group box, select the desired billing type range. For this exercise select all

4. In the *Select Date* group box, enter the desired date range and mark the desired options. The default is set with today's date, change the date if different.

5. In the *Select Totals* group box, check the desired options: For this exercise select MTD and YTD totals and include provider totals.

6. In the *Select Report Type* group box, check the desired options: For this exercise select *Chronological, Deposit Slip* (option ALL), *Daily Collections* (options ALL)

7. Click **OK** to send the report to the Batch Processor and return to the Office Manager

Print reports in the batch processor

To print reports you have sent to the Batch Processor

1. Select the report in the Batch Processor.

2. Click the **Print Report(s)** button.

           Chapter **17** Bookkeeping Procedures: Accounts Receivable

Delete reports from the batch processor

When reports are no longer needed it will be necessary to clear them from the Batch Processor.

1. Select the report in the Batch Processor.

2. Click the **Delete Report(s)** button. The Delete Options dialog appears.

3. In the *Delete* group box, mark the desired option.

4. Click **OK**

Dentrix Application

Scenario: As part of your daily routine, print out a copy of the Appointment Book for each operatory and a route slip for the patients you have scheduled (Jana Rogers, Angelica Green, Holly Barry, and Lynn Bacca, or others). At the end of each appointment, check out the patient by posting scheduled work, scheduling the next appointment, posting payments, and printing an insurance claim and walkout statement. At the end of the day generate a Day Sheet Report, Deposit Slip, and a Daily Collections Report.

At the end of this exercise you will have:

1. Printed a copy of the Appointment Book view.

2. Generated route slips for Jana Rogers, Angelica Green, Holly Barry, and Lynn Bacca, or other patients.

3. Scheduled the next appointment for each patient, using the information in each treatment plan.

4. Collected payments.

5. Printed an insurance claim form for each patient with insurance information.

6. Printed a walkout statement (Statement of Services Rendered) for each patient.

7. Printed a Day Sheet Report, Deposit Slip, and a Daily Collections Report.

Payment information
Jana Rogers
Payment (cash) .... $ 75.00 (check)
Angelica Green
Payment .... $125.00 (check)
Holly Barry
Payment (credit card) .... per financial agreement
Senior Citizen Discount .... per financial agreement
Lynn Bacca
Payment (cash) .... $ 50.00

Employment Strategies

LEARNING OBJECTIVES

1. List career opportunities for administrative dental assistants.
2. Identify and explain the steps to be followed in developing an employment strategy. Discuss the function of each step, including:
   - Construct a high-quality resume and cover letter.
   - Identify the avenues of where to look for employment.
   - Explain the function of a personal career portfolio and discuss its advantages.
   - Identify and respond to common interview questions.
   - Explain the proper way to accept and leave a job.

INTRODUCTION

Hundreds of jobs are waiting for the right person to fill them. The hiring decision is based on the ability of the prospective employee to successfully present himself or herself. Convincing the employer that you are the best person for the job is not easy. The process begins with a self-study and ends with a personal interview. Along the way, you will identify career options, answer questions about yourself, research possible employment opportunities, produce a quality resume, construct a letter of introduction, complete an application, and prepare mentally and physically for an interview.

EXERCISES

1. List the career opportunities for an administrative dental assistant.

_____

_____

_____

_____

_____

2. List and state the purpose of the steps involved in developing employment strategies.

_____

_____

_____

_____

_____

3. Describe the function of a personal career portfolio.

_____

_____

_____

_____

4. List the components of a personal career portfolio.

_____

_____

_____

_____

_____

5. List the components of a quality resume.

_____

_____

_____

_____

_____

_____

6. List the various avenues that may lead to employment.

_____

_____

_____

_____

_____

_____

ACTIVITY EXERCISES

7. Select a resume style (a chronological resume, a functional resume, or a hybrid resume) and produce a high-quality resume.

8. Write a cover letter.

DENTAL PRACTICE PROCEDURAL MANUAL PROJECT

Continue developing your procedural manual. Suggested components included in Chapter 18

■ Hiring

■ Reviews and Evaluations

■ Termination Procedures

DENTAL PRACTICE PROCEDURAL MANUAL PROJECT (OPTIONAL)

Continue working on your Dental Practice Procedural Manual (see Workbook Chapter 6 for details).
Suggested activities:

■ Team meeting

■ Review timeline

■ Review Group research and writing assignments

■ Complete research and writing assignments for this chapter

■ Review and revise completed sections of the manual

■ Individual journal entries

Appendix: Patient Paperwork

Jana Rogers

Canyon View Dental Associates
4546 North Avery Way
Canyon View, CA 91783
Telephone (987) 654-3210

Thank you for selecting our dental healthcare team!
We always strive to provide you with the best possible dental care.
To help us meet all your dental healthcare needs, please fill out this form completely.
Please let us know if you have any questions.

Patient Information (CONFIDENTIAL)

Patient # _____
Soc. Sec. # _____
Date _____

Name _____ Birthdate _____ Home Phone _____
Address _____ City _____ State _____ Zip _____
Check Appropriate Box: ☐ Minor ☐ Single ☐ Married ☐ Divorced ☐ Widowed ☐ Separated
Patient's or Parent's Employer _____ Work Phone _____
Business Address _____ City _____ State _____ Zip _____
Spouse or Parent's Name _____ Employer _____ Work Phone _____
If Patient is a Student, Name of School/College _____ City _____ State _____ Zip _____
Whom May We Thank for Referring you? _____
Person to Contact in Case of Emergency _____ Phone _____

Responsible Party

Name of Person Responsible for this Account _____
Relationship to Patient _____
Address _____ Home Phone _____
Driver's License # _____ Birthdate _____ Financial Information _____
Employer _____ Work Phone _____
Is this Person Currently a Patient in our Office? ☐ Yes ☐ No
Cell Phone _____
Email Address _____

Insurance Information

Name of Insured _____
Relationship to Patient _____
Birthdate _____ Social Security # _____ Date Employed _____
Name of Employer _____ Work Phone _____
Address of Employer _____ City _____ State _____ Zip _____
Insurance Company _____ Group # _____ Union or Local # _____
Ins. Co. Address _____ City _____ State _____ Zip _____
How Much is your Deductible? _____ How much have you met? _____ Max. Annual Benefit _____

DO YOU HAVE ANY ADDITIONAL INSURANCE? ☐ Yes ☐ NO IF YES, COMPLETE THE FOLLOWING

Name of Insured _____
Relationship to Patient _____
Birthdate _____ Social Security # _____ Date Employed _____
Name of Employer _____ Work Phone _____
Address of Employer _____ City _____ State _____ Zip _____
Insurance Company _____ Group # _____ Union or Local # _____
Ins. Co. Address _____ City _____ State _____ Zip _____
How Much is your Deductible? _____ How much have you met? _____ Max. Annual Benefit _____

I attest to the accuracy of the information on this page.

Patient's or guardian's signature _____ Date _____

REGISTRATION

These forms are intended for student use only

Jana Rogers

Canyon View Dental Associates
4546 North Avery Way
Canyon View, CA 91783
Telephone (987) 654-3210

Patient's name _____   Date of birth _____

Chief dental complaint		ORAL HYGIENE ☐EXCELLENT ☐GOOD ☐FAIR ☐POOR

	ORAL HYGIENE	☐EXCELLENT	☐GOOD	☐FAIR	☐POOR
Chief dental complaint	CALCULUS	☐NONE	☐LITTLE	☐MODERATE	☐HEAVY
	PLAQUE	☐NONE	☐LITTLE	☐MODERATE	☐HEAVY
Blood pressure Pulse	GINGIVAL BLEEDING		☐LOCALIZED	☐GENERAL	☐NONE
	PERIO EXAM ☐YES ☐NO				

Oral habits

New patient current restorations and missing teeth

Existing illness/current drugs

Allergies

Oral, soft tissue examination

	Description of any problem
Pharynx	
Tonsils	
Soft palate	
Hard palate	
Tongue	
Floor of mouth	
Buccal mucosa	
Lips skin	
Lymph nodes	
Occlusion	

Crown and bridge

Tooth #	Date placed	Condition

TMJ evaluation

Right	☐ Crepitus	☐ Snapping/popping
Left	☐ Crepitus	☐ Snapping/popping
Tenderness to palpation:		
TMJ	☐ Right	☐ Left
Muscles		
Deviation on closing	RMM	LMM
Needa further TMJ evaluation ☐ Yes ☐ No		
If yes, use TMJ evaluation form		

Extractions

Tooth #	Date extracted

Existing Prosthesis

Max.	Date placed:	Condition:
Min.	Date placed:	Condition:

Date _____

CLINICAL EXAMINATION

These forms are intended for student use only

Jana Rogers

Canyon View Dental Associates
4546 North Avery Way
Canyon View, CA 91783
Telephone (987) 654-3210

| | | | | | | |

Medical alert _____

Patient's name _____ Date of birth _____

Date	Tooth/ Surface	Time/ Units	Procedure code	Estimated fee	Treatment	Dr.	Asst./HYG.	Date completed

TREATMENT PLAN

These forms are intended for student use only

Jana Rogers

Canyon View Dental Associates
4546 North Avery Way
Canyon View, CA 91783
Telephone (987) 654-3210

⌐ ⌐ ⌐ ⌐ ⌐ ⌐ ⌐
PATIENT NUMBER

PATIENT'S NAME _____
                    Last   First   Initial

I _____ have had my treatment plan and options explained to me and hereby authorize this treatment to be performed by Dr. _____

Patient's Signature _____ Date _____
(Parent or Guardian MUST sign if patient is a minor)

I also understand that the cost of this treatment is as follows and that the method of paying for the same will be:

Total (Partial) estimate of treatment	$_____
Less:	
Initial Payment	—_____
Insurance Estimate If Applicable	—_____
Other _____	—_____
Balance of Estimate Due	$_____

Terms: Monthly Payment $ _____ over a _____ month period.

PLEASE CONTACT THE BUSINESS OFFICE IF YOU ARE UNABLE TO MEET YOUR FINANCIAL OBLIGA-TION

The truth in lending Law enacted in 1969 serves to inform the borrowers and installment purchasers of the true Annual Interest charged on the amounts financed. This law applies to this office whenever the office extends the courtesy of Installment Payments to our patients, even when no finance charge is made.

The signature below indicate a mutual understanding of the ESTIMATE for treatment and the acceptable schedule of payment as noted.

Today's Date _____
                          Signature of Responsible Party

_____
        Financial Advisor   Phone Number

Note: THIS IS AN ESTIMATE ONLY, if treatment plan should change please request an amended estimate should it not be offered by our staff. This estimate is valid for 90 days from the date above IF treatment has not begun within that period. A patient's voluntary termination of treatment makes this agreement invalid.

FINANCIAL ARRANGEMENTS

These forms are intended for student use only

Canyon View Dental Associates
4546 North Avery Way
Canyon View, CA 91783
Telephone (987) 654-3210

Thank you for selecting our dental healthcare team!
We always strive to provide you with the best possible dental care.
To help us meet all your dental healthcare needs, please fill out this form completely.
Please let us know if you have any questions.

Patient Information (CONFIDENTIAL)

Patient # _____

Soc. Sec. # _____

Date _____

Name _____ Birthdate _____ Home Phone _____

Address _____ City _____ State _____ Zip _____

Check Appropriate Box: ☐ Minor ☐ Single ☐ Married ☐ Divorced ☐ Widowed ☐ Separated

Patient's or Parent's Employer _____ Work Phone _____

Business Address _____ City _____ State _____ Zip _____

Spouse or Parent's Name _____ Employer _____ Work Phone _____

If Patient is a Student, Name of School/College _____ City _____ State _____ Zip _____

Whom May We Thank for Referring you? _____

Person to Contact in Case of Emergency _____ Phone _____

Responsible Party

Name of Person Responsible for this Account _____ Relationship to Patient _____

Address _____ Home Phone _____

Driver's License # _____ Birthdate _____ Financial Information _____

Employer _____ Work Phone _____

Is this Person Currently a Patient in our Office? ☐ Yes ☐ No

Cell Phone _____

Email Address _____

Insurance Information

Name of Insured _____ Relationship to Patient _____

Birthdate _____ Social Security # _____ Date Employed _____

Name of Employer _____ Work Phone _____

Address of Employer _____ City _____ State _____ Zip _____

Insurance Company _____ Group # _____ Union or Local # _____

Ins. Co. Address _____ City _____ State _____ Zip _____

How Much is your Deductible? _____ How much have you met? _____ Max. Annual Benefit _____

DO YOU HAVE ANY ADDITIONAL INSURANCE? ☐ Yes ☐ NO IF YES, COMPLETE THE FOLLOWING

Name of Insured _____ Relationship to Patient _____

Birthdate _____ Social Security # _____ Date Employed _____

Name of Employer _____ Work Phone _____

Address of Employer _____ City _____ State _____ Zip _____

Insurance Company _____ Group # _____ Union or Local # _____

Ins. Co. Address _____ City _____ State _____ Zip _____

How Much is your Deductible? _____ How much have you met? _____ Max. Annual Benefit _____

I attest to the accuracy of the information on this page.

Patient's or guardian's signature _____ Date _____

REGISTRATION

These forms are intended for student use only

Alicia Green

Canyon View Dental Associates
4546 North Avery Way
Canyon View, CA 91783
Telephone (987) 654-3210

Referred by_____ How would you rate the condition of your mouth? ☐ Excellent ☐ Good ☐ Fair ☐ Poor
Previous Dentist _____ How long have you been a patient?_____ Months/Years
Date of most recent dental exam _____/_____/_____ Date of most recent x-rays _____/_____/_____
Date of most recent treatment (other than a cleaning) _____/_____/_____
I routinely see my dentist every: ☐ 3 mo. ☐ 4 mo. ☐ 6 mo. ☐ 12 mo. ☐ Not routinely

WHAT IS YOUR IMMEDIATE CONCERN? _____

PLEASE ANSWER YES OR NO TO THE FOLLOWING: YES   NO

PERSONAL HISTORY

1. Are you fearful of dental treatment? How fearful, on a scale of 1 (least) to 10 (most) [___] _____ ☐ ☐
2. Have you had an unfavorable dental experience? _____ ☐ ☐
3. Have you ever had complications from past dental treatment? _____ ☐ ☐
4. Have you ever had trouble getting numb or had any reactions to local anesthetic? _____ ☐ ☐
5. Did you ever have braces, orthodontic treatment or had your bite adjusted? _____ ☐ ☐
6. Have you had any teeth removed? _____ ☐ ☐

SMILE CHARACTERISTICS

7. Is there anything about the appearance of your teeth that you would like to change? _____ ☐ ☐
8. Have you ever whitened (bleached) your teeth? _____ ☐ ☐
9. Have you felt uncomfortable or self conscious about the appearance of your teeth? _____ ☐ ☐
10. Have you been disappointed with the appearance of previous dental work? _____ ☐ ☐

BITE AND JAW JOINT

11. Do you have problems with your jaw joint? (pain, sounds, limited opening, locking, popping) _____ ☐ ☐
12. Do you / would you have any problems chewing gum? _____ ☐ ☐
13. Do you / would you have any problems chewing bagels, baguettes, protein bars, or other hard foods? _____ ☐ ☐
14. Have your teeth changed in the last 5 years, become shorter, thinner or worn? _____ ☐ ☐
15. Are your teeth crowding or developing spaces? _____ ☐ ☐
16. Do you have more than one bite and squeeze to make your teeth fit together? _____ ☐ ☐
17. Do you chew ice, bite your nails, use your teeth to hold objects, or have any other oral habits? _____ ☐ ☐
18. Do you clench your teeth in the daytime or make them sore? _____ ☐ ☐
19. Do you have any problems with sleep or wake up with an awareness of your teeth? _____ ☐ ☐
20. Do you wear or have you ever worn a bite appliance? _____ ☐ ☐

TOOTH STRUCTURE

21. Have you had any cavities within the past 3 years? _____ ☐ ☐
22. Does the amount of saliva in your mouth seem too little or do you have difficulty swallowing any food? _____ ☐ ☐
23. Do you feel or notice any holes (i.e. pitting, craters) on the biting surface of your teeth? _____ ☐ ☐
24. Are any teeth sensitive to hot, cold, biting, sweets, or avoid brushing any part of your mouth? _____ ☐ ☐
25. Do you have grooves or notches on your teeth near the gum line? _____ ☐ ☐
26. Have you ever broken teeth, chipped teeth, or had a toothache or cracked filling? _____ ☐ ☐
27. Do you get food caught between any teeth? _____ ☐ ☐

GUM AND BONE

28. Do your gums bleed when brushing or flossing? _____ ☐ ☐
29. Have you ever been treated for gum disease or been told you have lost bone around your teeth? _____ ☐ ☐
30. Have you ever noticed an unpleasant taste or odor in your mouth? _____ ☐ ☐
31. Is there anyone with a history of periodontal disease in your family? _____ ☐ ☐
32. Have you ever experienced gum recession? _____ ☐ ☐
33. Have you ever had any teeth become loose on their own (without an injury), or do you have difficulty eating an apple? _____ ☐ ☐
34. Have you experienced a burning sensation in your mouth? _____ ☐ ☐

Patient's Signature _____ Date_____

Doctor's Signature _____ Date_____

DENTAL HISTORY

These forms are intended for student use only

Alicia Green

Canyon View Dental Associates
4546 North Avery Way
Canyon View, CA 91783
Telephone (987) 654-3210

MEDICAL HISTORY

Patient Name _____ Nickname _____ Age _____
Name of Physician/and their specialty _____
Most recent physical examination _____ Purpose _____
What is your estimate of your general health? ☐Excellent ☐Good ☐Fair ☐Poor

DO YOU HAVE or HAVE YOU EVER HAD: YES   NO

1. hospitalization for illness or injury _____ ☐ ☐
2. an allergic reaction to
   - ☐ aspirin, ibuprofen, acetaminophen, codeine
   - ☐ penicillin
   - ☐ erythromycin
   - ☐ tetracycline
   - ☐ sulpha
   - ☐ local anesthetic
   - ☐ fluoride
   - ☐ metals (nickel, gold, silver, _____)
   - ☐ latex
   - ☐ other _____
3. heart problems, or cardiac stent within the last six months __ ☐ ☐
4. history of infective endocarditis _____ ☐ ☐
5. artificial heart valve, repaired heart defect (PFO) _____ ☐ ☐
6. pacemaker or implantable defibrillator _____ ☐ ☐
7. artificial prosthesis (heart valve or joints) _____ ☐ ☐
8. rheumatic or scarlet fever _____ ☐ ☐
9. high or low blood pressure _____ ☐ ☐
10. a stroke (taking blood thinners) _____ ☐ ☐
11. anemia or other blood disorder _____ ☐ ☐
12. prolonged bleeding due to a slight cut (INR > 3.5) _____ ☐ ☐
13. emphysema, sarcoidosis _____ ☐ ☐
14. tuberculosis _____ ☐ ☐
15. asthma _____ ☐ ☐
16. breathing or sleep problems (i.e. snoring, sinus) _____ ☐ ☐
17. kidney disease _____ ☐ ☐
18. liver disease _____ ☐ ☐
19. jaundice _____ ☐ ☐
20. thyroid, parathyroid disease, or calcium deficiency _____ ☐ ☐
21. hormone deficiency _____ ☐ ☐
22. high cholesterol or taking statin drugs _____ ☐ ☐
23. diabetes (HbA1c = _____) _____ ☐ ☐
24. stomach or duodenal ulcer _____ ☐ ☐
25. digestive disorders (i.e. gastric reflux) _____ ☐ ☐

                                                            YES   NO
26. osteoporosis/osteopenia (i.e. taking bisphosphonates) __ ☐ ☐
27. arthritis _____ ☐ ☐
28. glaucoma _____ ☐ ☐
29. contact lenses _____ ☐ ☐
30. head or neck injuries _____ ☐ ☐
31. epilepsy, convulsions (seizures) _____ ☐ ☐
32. neurologic problems (attention deficit disorder) _____ ☐ ☐
33. viral infections and cold sores _____ ☐ ☐
34. any lumps or swelling in the mouth _____ ☐ ☐
35. hives, skin rash, hay fever _____ ☐ ☐
36. venereal disease _____ ☐ ☐
37. hepatitis (type ___) _____ ☐ ☐
38. HIV / AIDS _____ ☐ ☐
39. tumor, abnormal growth _____ ☐ ☐
40. radiation therapy _____ ☐ ☐
41. chemotherapy _____ ☐ ☐
42. emotional problems _____ ☐ ☐
43. psychiatric treatment _____ ☐ ☐
44. antidepressant medication _____ ☐ ☐
45. alcohol / drug dependency _____ ☐ ☐

ARE YOU:
46. presently being treated for any other illness _____ ☐ ☐
47. aware of a change in your general health _____ ☐ ☐
48. taking medication for weight management (i.e. fen-phen) ☐ ☐
49. taking dietary supplements _____ ☐ ☐
50. often exhausted or fatigued _____ ☐ ☐
51. subject to frequent headaches _____ ☐ ☐
52. a smoker or smoked previously _____ ☐ ☐
53. considered a touchy person _____ ☐ ☐
54. often unhappy or depressed _____ ☐ ☐
55. FEMALE - taking birth control pills _____ ☐ ☐
56. FEMALE - pregnant _____ ☐ ☐
57. MALE - prostate disorders _____ ☐ ☐

Describe any current medical treatment, impending surgery, or other treatment that may possibly affect your dental treatment.

_____

List all medications, supplements, and or vitamins taken within the last two years

Drug	Purpose		Drug	Purpose

Ask for an additional sheet if you are taking more than 6 medications

PLEASE ADVISE US IN THE FUTURE OF ANY CHANGE IN YOUR MEDICAL HISTORY OR ANY MEDICATIONS YOU MAY BE TAKING.

Patient's Signature _____ Date _____
Doctor's Signature _____ Date _____

MEDICAL HISTORY

These forms are intended for student use only

Alicia Green

Canyon View Dental Associates
4546 North Avery Way
Canyon View, CA 91783
Telephone (987) 654-3210

Patient's name _____   Date of birth _____

Chief dental complaint		ORAL HYGIENE	☐ EXCELLENT	☐ GOOD	☐ FAIR	☐ POOR
		CALCULUS	☐ NONE	☐ LITTLE	☐ MODERATE	☐ HEAVY
		PLAQUE	☐ NONE	☐ LITTLE	☐ MODERATE	☐ HEAVY
Blood pressure Pulse		GINGIVAL BLEEDING		☐ LOCALIZED	☐ GENERAL	☐ NONE
		PERIO EXAM	☐ YES	☐ NO		

Oral habits

Existing illness/current drugs

Allergies

New patient current restorations and missing teeth

Oral, soft tissue examination

	Description of any problem
Pharynx	
Tonsils	
Soft palate	
Hard palate	
Tongue	
Floor of mouth	
Buccal mucosa	
Lips skin	
Lymph nodes	
Occlusion	

Crown and bridge

Tooth #	Date placed	Condition

TMJ evaluation

Right	☐ Crepitus	☐ Snapping/popping
Left	☐ Crepitus	☐ Snapping/popping
Tenderness to palpation:		
TMJ	☐ Right	☐ Left
Muscles		
Deviation on closing RMM LMM		
Needa further TMJ evaluation ☐ Yes ☐ No		
If yes, use TMJ evaluation form		

Extractions

Tooth #	Date extracted

Existing Prosthesis

Max.	Date placed:	Condition:
Min.	Date placed:	Condition:

Date _____

CLINICAL EXAMINATION

These forms are intended for student use only

143

Alicia Green

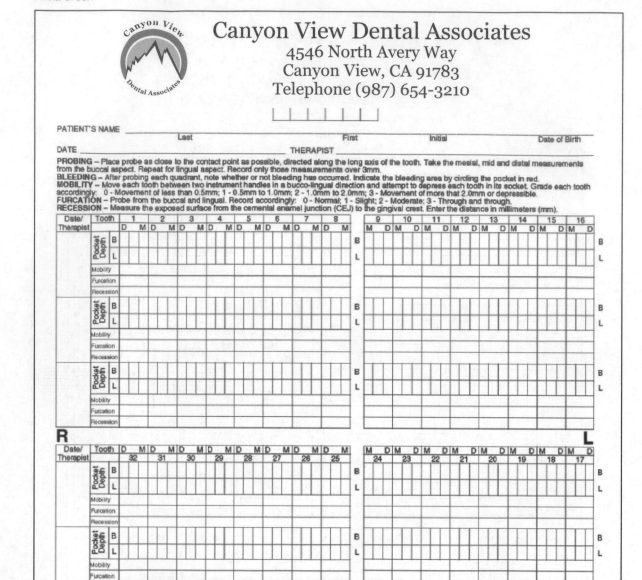

Canyon View Dental Associates
4546 North Avery Way
Canyon View, CA 91783
Telephone (987) 654-3210

| | | | | | | |

PATIENT'S NAME _____
Last   First   Initial   Date of Birth

DATE _____ THERAPIST _____

PROBING – Place probe as close to the contact point as possible, directed along the long axis of the tooth. Take the mesial, mid and distal measurements from the buccal aspect. Repeat for lingual aspect. Record only those measurements over 3mm.
BLEEDING – After probing each quadrant, note whether or not bleeding has occurred. Indicate the bleeding area by circling the pocket in red.
MOBILITY – Move each tooth between two instrument handles in a bucco-lingual direction and attempt to depress each tooth in its socket. Grade each tooth accordingly: 0 - Movement of less than 0.5mm; 1 - 0.5mm to 1.0mm; 2 - 1.0mm to 2.0mm; 3 - Movement of more that 2.0mm or depressible.
FURCATION – Probe from the buccal and lingual. Record accordingly: 0 - Normal; 1 - Slight; 2 - Moderate; 3 - Through and through.
RECESSION – Measure the exposed surface from the cemental enamel junction (CEJ) to the gingival crest. Enter the distance in millimeters (mm).

R   L

Enter highest POCKET DEPTH score in appropriate box	☐ Any pocket depth reading from 3 to 5mm, read below	☐ Any pocket depth reading over 5mm, read below
Enter highest MOBILITY SCORE in appropriate box	☐ Any mobility of 1, read below	☐ Any mobility of 2 or 3, read below

BLEEDING
☐ When any bleeding upon probing is noted, read below

INSTRUMENTS FOR TREATMENT SELECTION
Locate square containing score farthest to the right and follow treatment, listed below.

Gingivitis
☐ Explanation of periodontal disease.

A. Hygienist Treatment
 1. Oral Hygiene Instruction
 2. Prophylaxis

Moderate Periodontitis
OPTION 1
A. Dentist or Hygienist Treatment
 1. Oral Hygiene Instruction
 2. Periodontal Root Planing
 3. Occlusal Analysis
 4. Maintenance Recall
OPTION 2
B. Referral to Periodontist

Advanced Periodontitis
OPTION 1
A. Referral to Periodontist
OPTION 2
B. Dentist Treatment
 1. Oral Hygiene Instruction
 2. Periodontal Root Planing
 3. Occlusal Analysis
 4. Periodontal Surgery
 5. Splinting
 6. Maintenance Recall

PERIODONTAL SCREENING EXAMINATION

These forms are intended for student use only

Alicia Green

Canyon View Dental Associates
4546 North Avery Way
Canyon View, CA 91783
Telephone (987) 654-3210

Medical alert _____

Patient's name _____ Date of birth _____

	A	B	C	D	E	F	G	H	I	J	
R											L
	T	S	R	Q	P	O	N	M	L	K	

1	2	3	4	5	6	7	8	9	10	11	12	13	14	15	16
R															L
32	31	30	29	28	27	26	25	24	23	22	21	20	19	18	17

Date	Tooth/Surface	Time/Units	Procedure code	Estimated fee	Treatment	Dr. Asst./HYG.	Date completed

TREATMENT PLAN

These forms are intended for student use only

Canyon View Dental Associates
4546 North Avery Way
Canyon View, CA 91783
Telephone (987) 654-3210

PATIENT NUMBER

PATIENT'S NAME _____

            Last   First   Initial

I _____ have had my treatment plan and options explained to me and hereby authorize this treatment to be performed by Dr. _____

Patient's Signature _____ Date _____
(Parent or Guardian MUST sign if patient is a minor)

I also understand that the cost of this treatment is as follows and that the method of paying for the same will be:

Total (Partial) estimate of treatment	$ _____
Less:	
Initial Payment	— _____
Insurance Estimate if Applicable	— _____
Other _____	— _____
Balance of Estimate Due	$ _____

Terms: Monthly Payment $ _____ over a _____ month period.

PLEASE CONTACT THE BUSINESS OFFICE IF YOU ARE UNABLE TO MEET YOUR FINANCIAL OBLIGATION

The truth in lending Law enacted in 1969 serves to inform the borrowers and installment purchasers of the true Annual Interest charged on the amounts financed. This law applies to this office whenever the office extends the courtesy of Installment Payments to our patients, even when no finance charge is made.

The signature below indicate a mutual understanding of the ESTIMATE for treatment and the acceptable schedule of payment as noted.

Today's Date _____
                                      Signature of Responsible Party

_____
                     Financial Advisor   Phone Number

Note: THIS IS AN ESTIMATE ONLY, if treatment plan should change please request an amended estimate should it not be offered by our staff. This estimate is valid for 90 days from the date above IF treatment has not begun within that period. A patient's voluntary termination of treatment makes this agreement invalid.

FINANCIAL ARRANGEMENTS

These forms are intended for student use only

Holly Barry

Canyon View Dental Associates
4546 North Avery Way
Canyon View, CA 91783
Telephone (987) 654-3210

Thank you for selecting our dental healthcare team!
We always strive to provide you with the best possible dental care.
To help us meet all your dental healthcare needs, please fill out this form completely.
Please let us know if you have any questions.

Patient Information (CONFIDENTIAL)

Patient # _____
Soc. Sec. # _____
Date _____

Name _____ Birthdate _____   Home Phone _____
Address _____ City _____   State _____ Zip _____
Check Appropriate Box: ☐ Minor ☐ Single ☐ Married ☐ Divorced ☐ Widowed ☐ Separated
Patient's or Parent's Employer _____   Work Phone _____
Business Address _____ City _____   State _____ Zip _____
Spouse or Parent's Name _____ Employer_____   Work Phone_____
If Patient is a Student, Name of School/College _____ City _____ State_____ Zip _____
Whom May We Thank for Referring you? _____
Person to Contact in Case of Emergency _____   Phone _____

Responsible Party

Name of Person Responsible for this Account _____   Relationship to Patient _____
Address_____   Home Phone _____
Driver's License # _____ Birthdate _____   Financial Information _____
Employer_____   Work Phone _____
Is this Person Currently a Patient in our Office? ☐ Yes ☐ No   Cell Phone _____
                                                   Email Address _____

Insurance Information

Name of Insured_____   Relationship to Patient _____
Birthdate_____ Social Security # _____   Date Employed_____
Name of Employer _____   Work Phone _____
Address of Employer _____ City _____   State _____ Zip _____
Insurance Company_____ Group # _____   Union or Local # _____
Ins. Co. Address _____ City _____   State _____ Zip _____
How Much is your Deductible?_____ How much have you met?_____ Max. Annual Benefit _____

DO YOU HAVE ANY ADDITIONAL INSURANCE? ☐ Yes ☐ NO   IF YES, COMPLETE THE FOLLOWING

Name of Insured _____   Relationship to Patient _____
Birthdate _____ Social Security #_____   Date Employed _____
Name of Employer_____   Work Phone _____
Address of Employer_____ City_____   State _____ Zip_____
Insurance Company_____ Group #_____   Union or Local # _____
Ins. Co. Address_____ City_____   State_____ Zip_____
How Much is your Deductible? _____ How much have you met? _____ Max. Annual Benefit _____

I attest to the accuracy of the information on this page.

Patient's or guardian's signature _____ Date _____

REGISTRATION

These forms are intended for student use only

Canyon View Dental Associates
4546 North Avery Way
Canyon View, CA 91783
Telephone (987) 654-3210

Patient's name _____ Date of birth _____

Chief dental complaint		ORAL HYGIENE	☐EXCELLENT	☐GOOD	☐FAIR	☐POOR
		CALCULUS	☐NONE	☐LITTLE	☐MODERATE	☐HEAVY
		PLAQUE	☐NONE	☐LITTLE	☐MODERATE	☐HEAVY
Blood pressure Pulse		GINGIVAL BLEEDING		☐LOCALIZED ☐GENERAL	☐NONE
		PERIO EXAM	☐YES	☐NO	

Oral habits

Existing illness/current drugs

Allergies

New patient current restorations and missing teeth

Oral, soft tissue examination

	Description of any problem
Pharynx	
Tonsils	
Soft palate	
Hard palate	
Tongue	
Floor of mouth	
Buccal mucosa	
Lips skin	
Lymph nodes	
Occlusion	

Crown and bridge

Tooth #	Date placed	Condition

TMJ evaluation

Right	☐ Crepitus	☐ Snapping/popping
Left	☐ Crepitus	☐ Snapping/popping

Tenderness to palpation:

TMJ	☐ Right	☐ Left

Muscles

Deviation on closing   RMM   LMM

Needa further TMJ evaluation ☐ Yes ☐ No

If yes, use TMJ evaluation form

Extractions

Tooth #	Date extracted

Existing Prosthesis

Max.	Date placed:	Condition:
Min.	Date placed:	Condition:

Date _____

CLINICAL EXAMINATION

These forms are intended for student use only

Holly Barry

Canyon View Dental Associates
4546 North Avery Way
Canyon View, CA 91783
Telephone (987) 654-3210

Medical alert _____

Patient's name _____ Date of birth _____

Date	Tooth/Surface	Time/Units	Procedure code	Estimated fee	Treatment	Dr. Asst./HYG.	Date completed

TREATMENT PLAN

These forms are intended for student use only

Canyon View Dental Associates
4546 North Avery Way
Canyon View, CA 91783
Telephone (987) 654-3210

PATIENT NUMBER

PATIENT'S NAME _____

              Last   First   Initial

I _____ have had my treatment plan and options explained to me and hereby authorize this treatment to be performed by Dr. _____

Patient's Signature _____ Date _____
(Parent or Guardian MUST sign if patient is a minor)

I also understand that the cost of this treatment is as follows and that the method of paying for the same will be:

Total (Partial) estimate of treatment	$	_____
Less:		
Initial Payment	—	_____
Insurance Estimate if Applicable	—	_____
Other _____	—	_____
Balance of Estimate Due	$	_____

Terms: Monthly Payment $ _____ over a _____ month period.

PLEASE CONTACT THE BUSINESS OFFICE IF YOU ARE UNABLE TO MEET YOUR FINANCIAL OBLIGATION

The truth in lending Law enacted in 1969 serves to inform the borrowers and installment purchasers of the true Annual Interest charged on the amounts financed. This law applies to this office whenever the office extends the courtesy of Installment Payments to our patients, even when no finance charge is made.

The signature below indicate a mutual understanding of the ESTIMATE for treatment and the acceptable schedule of payment as noted.

Today's Date _____
                        Signature of Responsible Party

_____
         Financial Advisor   Phone Number

Note: THIS IS AN ESTIMATE ONLY, if treatment plan should change please request an amended estimate should it not be offered by our staff. This estimate is valid for 90 days from the date above IF treatment has not begun within that period. A patient's voluntary termination of treatment makes this agreement invalid.

FINANCIAL ARRANGEMENTS

These forms are intended for student use only

Lynn Bacca

Canyon View Dental Associates
4546 North Avery Way
Canyon View, CA 91783
Telephone (987) 654-3210

Thank you for selecting our dental healthcare team!
We always strive to provide you with the best possible dental care.
To help us meet all your dental healthcare needs, please fill out this form completely.
Please let us know if you have any questions.

Patient Information (CONFIDENTIAL)

Patient # _____
Soc. Sec. # _____
Date _____

Name _____ Birthdate _____ Home Phone _____
Address _____ City _____ State _____ Zip _____
Check Appropriate Box: ☐ Minor ☐ Single ☐ Married ☐ Divorced ☐ Widowed ☐ Separated
Patient's or Parent's Employer _____ Work Phone _____
Business Address _____ City _____ State _____ Zip _____
Spouse or Parent's Name _____ Employer _____ Work Phone _____
If Patient is a Student, Name of School/College _____ City _____ State _____ Zip _____
Whom May We Thank for Referring you? _____
Person to Contact in Case of Emergency _____ Phone _____

Responsible Party

Name of Person Responsible for this Account _____ Relationship to Patient _____
Address _____ Home Phone _____
Driver's License # _____ Birthdate _____ Financial Information _____
Employer _____ Work Phone _____
Is this Person Currently a Patient in our Office? ☐ Yes ☐ No
Cell Phone _____
Email Address _____

Insurance Information

Name of Insured _____ Relationship to Patient _____
Birthdate _____ Social Security # _____ Date Employed _____
Name of Employer _____ Work Phone _____
Address of Employer _____ City _____ State _____ Zip _____
Insurance Company _____ Group # _____ Union or Local # _____
Ins. Co. Address _____ City _____ State _____ Zip _____
How Much is your Deductible? _____ How much have you met? _____ Max. Annual Benefit _____

DO YOU HAVE ANY ADDITIONAL INSURANCE? ☐ Yes ☐ N0   IF YES, COMPLETE THE FOLLOWING

Name of Insured _____ Relationship to Patient _____
Birthdate _____ Social Security # _____ Date Employed _____
Name of Employer _____ Work Phone _____
Address of Employer _____ City _____ State _____ Zip _____
Insurance Company _____ Group # _____ Union or Local # _____
Ins. Co. Address _____ City _____ State _____ Zip _____
How Much is your Deductible? _____ How much have you met? _____ Max. Annual Benefit _____

I attest to the accuracy of the information on this page.

Patient's or guardian's signature _____ Date _____

REGISTRATION

These forms are intended for student use only

Appendix

Canyon View Dental Associates
4546 North Avery Way
Canyon View, CA 91783
Telephone (987) 654-3210

Patient's name _____ Date of birth _____

Chief dental complaint		ORAL HYGIENE	☐ EXCELLENT	☐ GOOD	☐ FAIR	☐ POOR
		CALCULUS	☐ NONE	☐ LITTLE	☐ MODERATE	☐ HEAVY
		PLAQUE	☐ NONE	☐ LITTLE	☐ MODERATE	☐ HEAVY
Blood pressure Pulse		GINGIVAL BLEEDING		☐ LOCALIZED ☐ GENERAL	☐ NONE	
		PERIO EXAM	☐ YES	☐ NO		

Oral habits

New patient current restorations and missing teeth

Existing illness/current drugs

Allergies

Oral, soft tissue examination

	Description of any problem
Pharynx	
Tonsils	
Soft palate	
Hard palate	
Tongue	
Floor of mouth	
Buccal mucosa	
Lips skin	
Lymph nodes	
Occlusion	

Crown and bridge

Tooth #	Date placed	Condition

TMJ evaluation

Right	☐ Crepitus	☐ Snapping/popping
Left	☐ Crepitus	☐ Snapping/popping
Tenderness to palpation:		
TMJ	☐ Right	☐ Left
Muscles		
Deviation on closing	RMM	LMM
Needa further TMJ evaluation ☐ Yes ☐ No		
If yes, use TMJ evaluation form		

Extractions

Tooth #	Date extracted

Existing Prosthesis

Max.	Date placed:	Condition:
Min.	Date placed:	Condition:

Date _____

CLINICAL EXAMINATION

These forms are intended for student use only

Lynn Bacca

Canyon View Dental Associates
4546 North Avery Way
Canyon View, CA 91783
Telephone (987) 654-3210

Medical alert _____

Patient's name _____ Date of birth _____

A	B	C	D	E	F	G	H	I	J

R   L

T	S	R	Q	P	O	N	M	L	K

1 2 3 4 5 6 7 8 9 10 11 12 13 14 15 16

R   L

32 31 30 29 28 27 26 25 24 23 22 21 20 19 18 17

Date	Tooth/ Surface	Time/ Units	Procedure code	Estimated fee	Treatment	Dr. Asst./HYG.	Date completed

TREATMENT PLAN

These forms are intended for student use only

Canyon View Dental Associates
4546 North Avery Way
Canyon View, CA 91783
Telephone (987) 654-3210

PATIENT NUMBER

PATIENT'S NAME _____

Last   First   Initial

I _____ have had my treatment plan and options explained to me and hereby
authorize this treatment to be performed by Dr. _____

Patient's Signature _____ Date _____
(Parent or Guardian MUST sign if patient is a minor)

I also understand that the cost of this treatment is as follows and that the method of paying for the same
will be:

Total (Partial) estimate of treatment	$	_____
Less:		
Initial Payment	—	_____
Insurance Estimate if Applicable	—	_____
Other _____	—	_____
Balance of Estimate Due	$	_____

Terms: Monthly Payment $ _____ over a _____ month period.

PLEASE CONTACT THE BUSINESS OFFICE IF YOU ARE UNABLE TO MEET YOUR FINANCIAL OBLIGA-
TION

The truth in lending Law enacted in 1969 serves to inform the borrowers and installment purchasers of the true Annual Interest charged on the
amounts financed. This law applies to this office whenever the office extends the courtesy of Installment Payments to our patients, even when no
finance charge is made.

The signature below indicate a mutual understanding of the ESTIMATE for treatment and the acceptable schedule of payment as noted.

Today's Date _____

Signature of Responsible Party

_____

Financial Advisor   Phone Number

Note: THIS IS AN ESTIMATE ONLY, if treatment plan should change please request an amended estimate should it not be offered by our staff.
This estimate is valid for 90 days from the date above IF treatment has not begun within that period. A patient's voluntary termination of treatment
makes this agreement invalid.

FINANCIAL ARRANGEMENTS

These forms are intended for student use only